WOMEN OF THE BIBLE

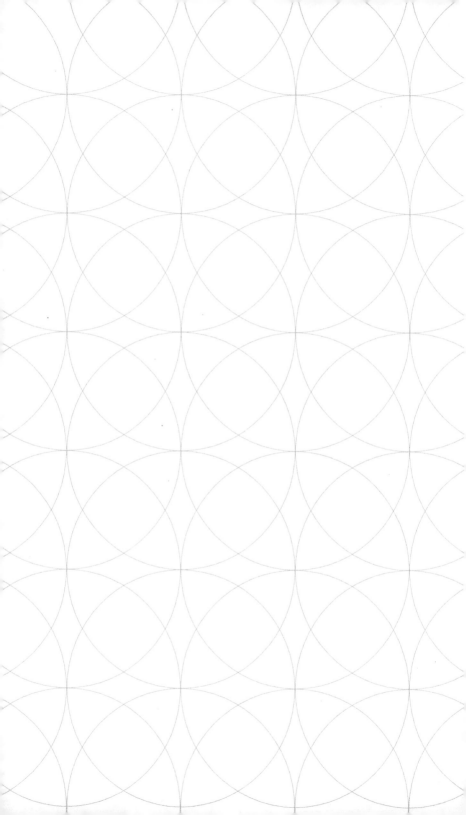

WOMEN
OF THE BIBLE

A 12-Week Bible Study for Christian Women

KIMBERLEE HERMAN, MSW, LCPC

ROCKRIDGE
PRESS

Interior and Cover Designer: Lori Cervone
Art Producer: Samantha Ulban
Editors: Samantha Holland and Mo Mozuch
Production Editor: Jael Fogle
Production Manager: Riley Hoffman

All images used under license © iStock.
Author photo courtesy of Chad Dahlquist.

Paperback ISBN: 978-1-63807-929-3
eBook ISBN: 978-1-63807-863-0
R0

———

This book is dedicated to my loving family: my husband, Dave, for being my biggest cheerleader, and our daughter, Madison, who gave me hugs and encouragement to keep me focused. They both gave me space to study and write this book, and I am most grateful. I am also so thankful to God, who held my hand through this process and helped me highlight the precious women who came before us.

———

Contents

Introduction

Welcome! I am so glad you are here. This book is written for all Christian women, no matter their denomination or background, who desire to learn how God called, utlized, helped, and taught women throughout the scriptures—women who, you'll see, are pretty similar to you and me in many ways. Throughout these pages, you will learn how women who are coping with all sorts of adversity can rise up when they are called to be a part of God's plans or His works. (Spoiler alert: We are all part of God's plans and works! See Ephesians 2:10.) The insights and revelation we can gather from these precious women's stories can encourage us to persevere, hold ourselves high, and know that even if we make decisions that are not the best, God can work through those choices (Romans 8:28).

I hope reading this book will be a meaningful experience for everyone interested in diving deeper into God's Word and applying it to their lives. This book is for those of you who want to learn more about the women of the Bible and how their stories relate to your own life and for those who want to be inspired in surprising ways. Do you prefer independent study or learning in a group setting? You can easily use this book for both. Check out the Group Study Guide on page 105 if you'd like to explore this book as a shared experience with others.

In the chapters that follow, we'll focus on 12 women from the Bible and their impact on our history of faith. Most of the women we'll be discussing are not perfect. They stumble, they make decisions that hurt others, and they are human—just like us. When we read their stories and think about their lives, we can relate to some of, if not all, their journeys. We'll see, again and again, that God does not condemn them for their wrong choices. Instead, He rescues, fixes, and adjusts the areas of their lives that need repairing. What sets these women apart is not that they are flawless, but that even in their imperfection, God works through them because God's plans are in action. The same is true for all of us.

Out of around 200 women in the Bible, we are focusing our attention on 12. The actions and words of these dozen women had a profound impact not only during their time but also today in what we can learn from them. I've selected these women to illustrate how throughout the centuries, God has chosen ordinary people from all social classes to do the unexpected despite their own mistakes and humanity. The women you're about to meet have very different personalities, live unique lives, and each brings a different perspective and view of the world and God.

We can learn so much from those who came before us. As a Christian counselor, I have talked with many women who struggle internally. Many battle depression because of negative internal self-talk. Others feel guilty because they are not perfect or because they made the wrong choices. They then stray from God because of this guilt. Self-criticism and bitterness creep in. None of us are perfect, so none of us are immune from falling into this thinking pattern. My clients have learned new thinking patterns through healing work, but I know many people do not seek help like they did. This book is not a substitute for professional counseling or medical treatment. I also believe understanding that God works through our imperfections to bring His divine plan into fruition can bring us tremendous peace and help us realize it is okay not to be perfect.

This realization brings me peace when I'm troubled. My prayer is that this book will usher a beautiful sense of peace into your own life, too. I am so delighted to take this journey with you!

How to Use This Bible Study

O ur study is organized into 12 weeklong sessions, each focusing on the life of one woman from the Bible. At the beginning of every week, you'll find an introduction and a list of scripture passages for the week to come. On the first day, read the introduction, then the day's assigned scripture, and then the commentary. Continue this practice of reading one passage and commentary every day. At the end of each day, if possible, conclude your study by considering the reflection questions intended to help you dive deeper into the meaning of each passage. On the final day, instead of a scriptural reading, you'll find a list of key insights to sum up the week's study. You'll also find a short roster of activities and challenges for you to try based on the week's readings.

The goal of this Bible study is for you to learn about the women in the Bible through their stories and to apply their lessons to your own life through the week's insights and action items. Try to incorporate this book into your daily routine, making time to do the reading and reflecting. Each day's reading assignment is brief, so it shouldn't take more than 15 minutes a day to read each Bible passage and the related commentary. But if you can find more time, especially for reflection, you'll likely have a more rewarding experience. If you are interested in using this guide in a group setting, turn to the Group Study Guide (page 105) for more information. There's also a list of resources in the back of the book with additional materials you may find useful. On the other hand, life can get crazy busy, so don't stress if you miss a day. Simply pick up where you left off and keep going. It is your journey. Make this study work for you and your schedule.

You will need the following materials:

1. This book.

2. A Bible of your choice, with both the Old and New Testament. This book uses the English Standard Version (ESV), but any version will work fine.

3. A pen or pencil and a notebook or journal to write in, or you can record audio responses on a phone or digital recorder. Although it is optional, I strongly recommend documenting your answers for the reflection questions, as well as notes and thoughts about the readings and anything else you'd like to keep track of during your study.

Are you ready? I am so excited for you to embark on your adventure with these 12 amazing women! Together we will follow in their footsteps and take steps forward in understanding their decisions and actions. We'll learn and hopefully be changed in some way by honoring God, ourselves, and the wisdom we can glean from women who walked in faith before us.

SARAI: WHAT'S IN A NAME?

Daily Readings

Day 1: Genesis 11:29–31, Genesis 12:1–20

Day 2: Genesis 16:1–16

Day 3: Genesis 17:15–21

Day 4: Genesis 18:1–15

Day 5: Genesis 20:1–18, Genesis 21:1–7, Hebrews 11:11

Day 6: Genesis 21:8–21, Galatians 4:22–31

Day 7: Reflect and Take Action

Sarai lives a challenging but rewarding life, full of shame, promises, frustration, and a birth that generations later ushers in Jesus. When we first meet Sarai (pronounced "Saw-rye"), she's a beautiful young woman whose name means "princess." As the first matriarch in the line of Jesus, her name hints at the coming of the One who would be called King of Kings (Revelation 17:14).

In Genesis, Sarai marries Abram. In Sarai's culture, not having a child brings shame to a husband and wife. Sarai is barren for most of her years, but God promises to bless her and her husband with a son. We'll see that Sarai finds it hard to be patient with God's timing.

When Sarai is 89, God meets with Abram. This meeting is when everything changes for Sarai. God gives them both new names. He also declares Sarai will give birth within a year, and she laughs in response. But God proclaims, "Is anything too hard for the Lord?"

This week, we will look into Sarai's heart and discover how God works through times of darkness and bitterness. Sarai teaches us that life can be challenging, but God's promises do not falter. We watch Sarai take matters into her own hands out of impatience then get angry at the result of her decisions. But God has her in His care and works through her choices and reactions.

Sarah, formerly Sarai, is known for her beauty, but even in the midst of ugliness we will see God's magnificent plan unfold through her.

| Day 1

The Beautiful Princess
Genesis 11:29–31, Genesis 12:1–20

God directs Abram and his family to move to Canaan, where He will abundantly bless them. Because of famine, Abram and Sarai live for a season in nearby Egypt, where there is food available. Sarai is very beautiful, and Abram is concerned that the ruler of Egypt, the Pharaoh, will kill Abram to get her. So they tell a lie of omission: Sarai and Abram declare they are siblings but keep silent about being married. (They were, in fact, half-siblings because they had the same father [Genesis 20:12]. It was how things were back then.) Pharaoh takes Sarai as a concubine, but God intervenes by afflicting Pharaoh's family with plagues. Pharaoh realizes Sarai is married and returns her to Abram.

Abram and Sarai do not trust God to protect them, so they rely on deception to try to avoid danger. Without this plan, her hope of having Abram's promised son will be stolen, and her shame at being childless will remain. Sarai is put in danger nonetheless. But through it all, hope survives. Like a princess in a fairy tale, Sarai is rescued by God.

FOR REFLECTION

1. Can you think of a time when you needed to tell a lie, like Sarai did, in order to protect a bigger truth? Did the lie help or hurt the situation? Would you do it again?

2. Sarai must have felt very frightened in Egypt. Think back to a time when you were afraid and uncertain. What did you do? What helped you get through your fear?

Day 2

Sarai's Plan
Genesis 16:1–16

Sarai and Abram have been in Canaan for 10 years, and they've been married for a long time without producing a child. As mentioned earlier, having a child was considered an essential duty for women to carry on their legacy and bring honor to their family and lineage.

Feeling the pressure, Sarai decides that because she is barren, her maidservant Hagar will bear the child that she can't. Sarai convinces Abram to go along with this idea.

Sarai gives Hagar to Abram to be his second wife. When Hagar conceives, she looks down at Sarai, so Sarai "dealt harshly with her." Hagar reacts to this mistreatment by running away. The shame, jealousy, and disappointment boiling inside Sarai are evident, but God's plan is still intact. He intervenes in Sarai's anger and has compassion for Hagar.

Sarai's impatience leads her to make a plan in a state of frustration. But God does not give His blessing over Abram's marriage to Hagar, so it is destined to fail. Sarai's desperate decision leads to an inherently unsustainable situation. When Sarai's emotions took over, God interceded.

1. Sarai is around 76 years old when she has the idea for Hagar to conceive with Abram. Why do you think she develops the plan at this time?

2. Have you ever agreed to a bad decision in desperate circumstances, like Abram? What happened?

3. Recall a time when you had to make a painful choice for what seemed like an important reason. How did you decide what to do? Did you regret it afterward? How did it change things?

Day 3

Sarah the Noblewoman
Genesis 17:15–21

Things take a sharp positive turn for Sarai. God tells Abram that Sarai is now to be called Sarah, which means "noblewoman." Abram's name is changed to Abraham, "father of many." God changes their names to usher in the promise He has for them, signifying a new season and a new purpose. Sarah will be appointed the first matriarch in the line of Jesus.

Until then, Abraham believes Ishmael, his son through Hagar, is the one chosen by God to bring forth "nations as numerous as the stars." Instead he learns that God is the God of the impossible: Sarah is 89 and Abraham 99 when they are told Sarah will carry the child of the promise and to name him Isaac.

God tells Abraham that he will bless Sarah twice. God is not only going to bless her with a son, but Sarah will also be the matriarch of nations, and kings will come through her. It is a huge promise of hope Sarah can hold on to—if she believes. Sometimes God's promises are too much for us to comprehend, as we will see tomorrow.

1. What do you think is the significance of changing Sarai's name to Sarah?

2. God surprises Abraham and Sarah with new names and a child at a late age. God can surprise us in many ways. What are the biggest surprises God has placed in your life?

Day 4

Sarah Laughs
Genesis 18:1–15

God unexpectedly visits Abraham's home with two companions. Abraham offers to serve them dinner outside. In those days, it was customary for the wife of the household to stay in the tent when guests were present (remember they are nomads, or tent dwellers). Sarah does not come out, but she can hear what Abraham and God are discussing. To her surprise, they are talking about her.

God reveals that Sarah will have a baby the following year. Sarah, who is 89 years old, laughs out loud at this idea and doubts what she hears. God hears her laugh. He reminds Abraham (and Sarah) that nothing is too difficult for Him to accomplish.

Certainly we can understand Sarah's reaction. The whole thing must have seemed ridiculous. How could she give birth at her age? God's plans make no sense to Sarah because He is promising the impossible; she could not help but laugh. But God shows us through Sarah that His plan will happen in His timing, not ours. What seems absurd to Sarah, what appears impossible to us, is never beyond God's reach.

FOR REFLECTION

1. Can you think of a time when you considered something to be ridiculous only to find out it was true? How did you handle it?

2. God Himself declares the child of Sarah and Abraham will be named Isaac (from day 3), which means "to laugh." Do you know the history behind your name? Is it meaningful to you? Why or why not? Is there anyone in your life whom you refer to with a nickname that holds special meaning?

Day 5

God to the Rescue (Again)!
Genesis 20:1–18, Genesis 21:1–7, Hebrews 11:11

Soon after God leaves their home, Sarah is again put into a perilous position. When they move to Gerar (modern-day Israel), Abraham is terrified that King Abimelech will kill him and take Sarah as his wife because she is still very beautiful. (Sound familiar?) Abraham falls back on his old lie and tells the king they are siblings. Sarah is taken away at 89 years old to be a wife to the king. Even Sarah, who will give birth to a nation, has to endure much hardship.

God intervenes again, telling the king in a dream that Sarah needs to return to Abraham. The king returns Sarah and, to make things right, gives them silver, servants, and animals. Sarah and Abraham leave richer than when they arrived.

And in God's perfect timing, He brings about the miracle that allows Sarah to conceive. She brings Isaac into the world. Knowing what his name means, Sarah is joyful believing that others will laugh with her when they hear her story of miracles, promises, and patience. Her son will be a reminder of Sarah's initial reaction to God's promise of the impossible.

FOR REFLECTION

1. Why do you think Abraham and Sarah lie to the king after God tells him His promise again? Can you think of a time when, faced with a recurring problem, you reverted to the same ineffective solution?

2. When fear makes it hard for you to trust in God, what do you do to remind yourself of His blessings?

Day 6

Sarah's Anger
Genesis 21:8–21, Galatians 4:22–31

We don't always act our best when defending our children. When Sarah witnesses Ishmael laughing at or mocking Isaac, she demands that Abraham send away Ishmael and his mother, Hagar. Abraham banishes them. When Hagar and Ishmael are out of water in the desert, Hagar cries out to God. God hears her and changes their lives. The Lord not only supplies water for them but also promises Hagar that Ishmael will father a great nation.

Galatians 4:22–31 discusses the differences between Sarah and Hagar. Hagar was an enslaved person while Sarah was a free woman. To this day, followers of Christ are considered children of Sarah, not children of Hagar. Jesus came through Sarah and brings freedom to His followers even to this day (Galatians 5:1).

And yet it's Sarah who acts badly here. Sarah does not think through to the consequences of her treatment of Hagar, which is what happens when we make decisions out of anger. We can take wisdom not just from considering Sarah's acts but also from what happened afterward. God shows us that despite Sarah's fury, He takes care of things by rescuing Hagar and Ishmael. Where we can be harsh, God is compassionate.

FOR REFLECTION

1. Sarah's anger gets the best of her when she sees Ishmael mocking Isaac. Most mothers can relate to protecting their children and losing it if a bully comes around. What kinds of things make you lose your cool? Is there a better way of handling things when you get angry?

2. What lesson can we learn from the fact that God hears and looks after Hagar when she is sent away by Sarah?

Day 7: Reflect and Take Action

KEY INSIGHTS

- Sarah is human and not beyond emotion. God intervenes with His compassion for Hagar and Ishmael when Sarah is not able to. But God does not abandon His promise. We can all have faith that God will not abandon us when we fall short.

- God names Isaac, which means "to laugh," before Sarah's reaction to the news that she will be pregnant. God knows our doubts and insecurities before we realize them. Although God's plan does allow for human error, we see in Sarah's story that God intervenes when she is impatient with Him. He is strong when she is weak.

ACTION ITEMS

Look up the meaning of your name. Does it resonate with you? Would you rather have another name? What is it?

Are there areas in your life that need rescuing by God? Pray and ask for wisdom and His help. Doing so often involves making new choices. Listen for His direction.

Write about moments in your life when you felt God took you in a different direction or brought a surprise to your life that changed things.

Hebrews 11:11 states that Sarah had faith in order to conceive. Mark 9:23 states anything is possible if you believe. Why do you think faith is so important? Do you believe miracles happen today? Why or why not? Discuss faith and miracles with a friend for a different perspective.

REBEKAH: SECURING THE BLESSING

Daily Readings

Day 1: Genesis 24:1–27

Day 2: Genesis 24:28–61

Day 3: Genesis 24:62–67, Genesis 25:19–28

Day 4: Genesis 26:1–13

Day 5: Genesis 27:1–29

Day 6: Genesis 27:30–46

Day 7: Reflect and Take Action

Rebekah's story begins soon after Sarah's ends, and it starts from an interesting perspective as she unknowingly answers a prayer from Abraham's emissary. Her act of kindness changes her life, signaling she's destined to be the bride of Isaac, the son of Abraham and Sarah.

Rebekah and Isaac are married, and Rebekah becomes pregnant. God tells expectant Rebekah the destinies of her twin sons, Jacob and Esau. Her strong faith in what God tells her is in stark contrast to the wavering faith of Sarah from last week's scripture. We see in Rebekah many traits we can aspire to: She's strong in her faith, hardworking, true to her word, modest, and proactive. These characteristics serve her and her family well—until a defining moment, involving Isaac, when she chooses deceit over prayer.

We learn from Rebekah that despite our best qualities, we can be lured into the false belief that it is our responsibility to "fix" something instead of bringing our concerns to God. Had Rebekah simply let God's will unfold, rather than relying on trickery to soothe her doubts, she may not have been separated from her favored son, Jacob, for the rest of her life. There is much wisdom to learn from Rebekah's strengths and weaknesses.

| Day 1

Prayer in Action
Genesis 24:1–27

Isaac is around 40 years old and needs a wife. Abraham does not want his son to marry a local Canaanite woman, and he cannot allow Isaac to return to his clan. Instead, Abraham sends his servant to the city of Nahor with strict orders to bring back a wife for Isaac. Abraham has faith that God has already selected a wife. When the servant arrives outside Nahor, he prays for specific signs to help him find the chosen woman. Everything is put in God's hands.

We see prayer in action as Rebekah's offer of water for Abraham's servant and his camels answers the servant's prayer request. Rebekah's generosity as she offers her home to this stranger and his helpers shows us that God looks at the hearts of people. He must have seen the kindness in her character and considered it in choosing her to join Abraham's family. Almost immediately after Rebekah offers water, she is rewarded in the form of gifts from Abraham's servant. But there will be greater rewards to come.

1. When was the last time a stranger asked for your help, even in a minor way? How did you respond? Have you ever regretted help-ing a stranger in need?

2. Abraham has faith that a wife was already selected for Isaac, but he also takes action to find her, rather than expecting God to deliver her to his door. In your own life, how do you know when to take action and when to leave the results to God?

Day 2

Handpicked by God
Genesis 24:28–61

You can feel the excitement of Abraham's servant as he meets Rebekah's family and insists on sharing his story and explaining his answered prayer. He has just traveled a very long distance, yet he postpones having a meal and rest so he can proclaim the goodness of God.

His instinct proves correct: Rebekah's family trusts that she is chosen. They allow the servant to take her back to Isaac. Immediately afterward, the servant gives thanks to God again, showing the impor-tance of putting God first.

Although Rebekah's family is reserved about her leaving right away, after discussing it, they ask her what she wants to do. She agrees to go immediately. Before Rebekah leaves, her family speaks a blessing over her, which foreshadows an important aspect of Rebekah's life that will be discussed later this week.

Consider that Rebekah does not hesitate to go, even though it means leaving her family and home behind and going into unknown territory. To possess such bravery, she, too, must feel God's plan all over this engagement. Walking out in faith, without doubt or questioning, is the wisdom we learn from Rebekah in this passage.

1. Rebekah immediately recognizes the good thing God has sent her way. Name something good in your life that you didn't appreciate at first.

2. When have you had Rebekah's kind of faith? What were the circumstances?

Day 3

The New Matriarch
Genesis 24:62–67, Genesis 25:19–28

The scripture describes the meeting of Isaac and Rebekah in a beautiful manner, with each seeing the other from afar and wondering, "Who is that?" We witness Rebekah's modesty as she veils herself before she meets her future husband (Genesis 24:63–65).

Rebekah is put into the role of the female head of the family right away by giving her the matriarchal tent of his mother, Sarah. They marry, Isaac loves her, and Rebekah brings him comfort while he is still mourning the death of his mother, Sarah.

The two have been married for about 20 years when Isaac prays for Rebekah to have children. Not knowing she has conceived twins, she asks God why she feels commotion in her womb. He gives her His prophecy about her babies: Her sons will become two nations, and the older will serve the younger.

Until now, Rebekah has seemed pretty perfect: strong in faith, modest, and a comfort to her husband. But one of the notable things we can learn from her, and the other women of the Bible, is that most of them are flawed. Just like us, their struggle can sometimes give way to their worst impulses, like we will see with Rebekah later in her story. It begins with choosing a favorite child.

1. What does it say about Rebekah that she goes God to ask what is going on in her pregnancy? How often do you turn to God when faced with something you don't understand?

2. Isaac favors Esau because he loves eating game, and Esau is a good hunter. Rebekah favors Jacob. This favoritism is going to lead to trouble. What do you think about parents having a favorite child? Is it ever okay?

Day 4

Laughing with Isaac
Genesis 26:1-13

This passage appears to take us back to before the twins were born, with parallels to the story of Isaac's parents, Abraham and Sarah. Isaac and Rebekah head south to Gerar (modern-day Israel) because of famine. God promises Isaac the same thing he did Abraham, that he will "multiply his offspring." This promise reminds us that the blessing Rebekah's family gave her when she left them will, in fact, come to pass.

Isaac and Rebekah run into another King Abimelech. As Abraham did before him, Isaac tells the king that he and Rebekah are siblings and not married. Again this ruse fails. The king sees Isaac and Rebekah together and realizes they are married. He sends her back to Isaac and warns everyone to stay away from them.

The repetition of this scenario reminds us that we learn from our parents and can even repeat their mistakes. Isaac has a profound experience with God, yet soon afterward he fears for his life and hides his relationship with Rebekah to try to protect himself. Learning to lean into God's promises, or calling out to God for help, could have kept them from creating the lie that angered the king and kept Rebekah out of a perilous position.

1. What personality traits and patterns have you inherited from your parents? Are there any you want to change? Are there any you are proud of?

2. What are your thoughts about maintaining a public persona that's different from who you are in private, whether it's concealing a relationship or keeping your personal life to yourself?

Day 5

Prophecy Unfolds
Genesis 27:1–29

This passage is what Rebekah is most known for, and it is not her finest moment. Remember what God told her when she was pregnant with the twins (Genesis 25:23)? Rebekah must remember those words when she hears Isaac, who is very old and blind, wanting to bless their older son, Esau. She decides to be proactive. Rebekah insists Jacob obey and follow her plan to trick Isaac into believing Jacob is Esau so Jacob will receive the blessing instead. We do not know if Isaac did not listen to God's plans for Jacob, if he has forgotten in his old age, or if Rebekah believes she is doing the right thing. In the end, she deceives Isaac, and because God is sovereign, He allows it to happen.

We all have gifts, and we can use them in different ways. Rebekah used her traits of faithfulness, hard work, and proactivity in her ploy. We can sometimes use great attributes for selfish gain or in misunderstanding God's Word. God will allow our plans because He gave us free will, but not all our plans fall in line with His (Proverbs 19:21).

1. Rebekah could have asked God for guidance or stepped back to let God handle His prophecy in His own time. Why do you think she did not do so? What can we learn from her deceptive actions?

2. Reflect on a time when you introduced a deception or falsehood into a relationship. What did it feel like? What was the result?

3. Rebekah believes she needs to make this blessing happen, based on what God told her when she was pregnant. But using deception is not the right way. What have you witnessed when others have misunderstood their role in the Word of God and created their own plan? What were the repercussions?

Day 6

The Fallout
Genesis 27:30–46

Everything begins to unravel in this passage. Esau is so angry that he was deceived and did not get his blessing that he threatens to kill Jacob. Rebekah believes Esau would murder his brother, so she sends Jacob away. Her children are in conflict, and Rebekah does not see her favored son again.

Rebekah is a strong woman who has faith in God's Word but tries to usher in His plan in her own way. As a consequence of her actions, Jacob is put in grave danger from Esau's wrath, and she is separated permanently from her favorite son. Despite all this, God was still able to work through Rebekah's poor choices, just like He does with us today. Rebekah leaves us with the wisdom of not leaning on our own understanding of God and His plans, as Proverbs 3:5–6 reminds us.

FOR REFLECTION

1. Have you ever really pushed yourself to get what you wanted, like Rebekah did? What happened?

2. After all the scheming, it does not appear that Rebekah sees Jacob again. What does that tell us about the importance of what she felt she needed to do? And about her family relationships? How do you feel about your family relationships? What would you do for them?

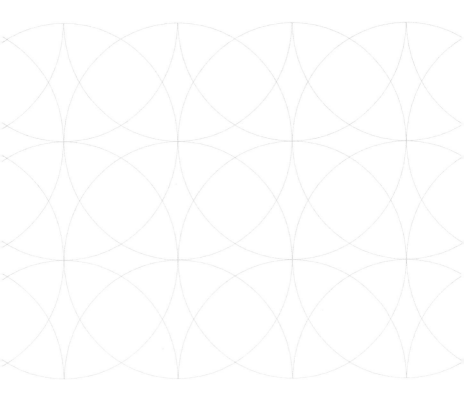

Day 7: Reflect and Take Action

KEY INSIGHTS

- The world calls it coincidence, but we understand it as God's plan when Rebekah is chosen to be Isaac's wife because she is there at just the right time for Abraham's servant to interact with her. Sometimes we can be an answer to someone's prayer without realizing it.

- Just like Sarai planned for Hagar to conceive Abram's child, Rebekah comes up with a questionable strategy for Jacob to receive a blessing. Both women take problems into their own hands without asking God for His help. We all are susceptible to doing the same thing because we are human. Remembering how Rebekah is separated from her son as a consequence can help us be humble and turn to God when making our decisions.

ACTION ITEMS

No one is perfect, even if they appear to be. What attributes do you like within yourself? What don't you like? Ask God to help you strengthen your good attributes and put away your challenging ones.

Find a board or card game you can play with your spouse or significant other to have fun, like Rebekah did with Isaac. If you are not in a relationship, host a game night for your friends. If you are stumped on games, a favorite in our house is Wits and Wagers.

Do you identify with any of Rebekah's positive characteristics of being courageous, adaptable, and modest? Are there any you aspire to? What changes could you make to develop those traits? Journal your thoughts.

LEAH: THE TRANSFORMED SISTER

Daily Readings

Day 1: Genesis 29:1–24

Day 2: Genesis 29:25–30

Day 3: Genesis 29:31

Day 4: Genesis 29:32–35

Day 5: Genesis 30:9–21

Day 6: Genesis 30:25–43, Genesis 31:1–55

Day 7: Reflect and Take Action

L eah is best known in conjunction with her sister, Rachel, because both sisters were married to Jacob. This week we are spending time with only Leah because she is the sister whose lineage brings us to Jesus. She is overlooked, unloved, jealous, and used by her father, but then she learns to praise God in her circumstances and is changed in her heart.

We first meet Leah after Jacob has been living with Laban, his mother Rebekah's brother, for one month. Jacob falls in love with Leah's sister, Rachel, who is considered the beautiful one. Leah comes into the story as a quiet sideline character, hardly noticed, but will soon be in the spotlight. We will see Leah blossom as her devotion to God transforms her heart.

Leah's story shows us that although we can feel overlooked and not as important as others, God does not see us that way. He can use ordinary people to do great things. In addition, we can admire Leah because even though she doesn't get the love she wants from Jacob, she doesn't turn bitter. Instead, she learns to focus on the blessings in her life. Leah's account is a great reminder for us to turn to God when things do not go the way we want them to.

Day 1

The Quiet Sister
Genesis 29:1–24

Our story begins when Jacob flees his home to get away from his furious brother, Esau, and the deception he and his mother, Rebekah, created. Isaac does not send any flocks or wealth with Jacob, so he cannot offer any dowry to his uncle Laban (Rebekah's brother) for a wife. Instead, Jacob offers to work seven years to marry Rachel (Leah's sister).

One month after Jacob's arrival, we meet Leah, the older, "weak eyed" (tender or sad) sister. Jacob, in love with Rachel, has no interest in Leah. After seven years Laban throws a wedding feast. Jacob believes he is marrying Rachel. But after the feast, Leah is brought to Jacob at night, when it is dark and the substitution will go unnoticed. Intimacy follows, and the act makes them married.

Leah's father puts her in a situation most of us would be mortified to play out: She is made to go into Jacob's bed pretending she is Rachel. Although it appears that Leah wants to marry Jacob, this situation is awful.

She chooses to put her own feelings aside, does not complain about a situation she cannot control, and accepts the circumstances she is given.

FOR REFLECTION

1. Leah is put into an uncomfortable situation by her father, who has absolute authority in her home because of the culture at the time. Despite the unfairness, she handles herself with grace. Does someone have authority in your life (maybe your boss)? How do you handle the situation when you're asked to do something that seems unfair?

2. Jacob deceives his father, Isaac, who cannot see, and is himself deceived in darkness. Can you recall a time when someone treated you badly, and you realized you'd done the same thing to someone else?

Day 2

Unrequited Love
Genesis 29:25–30

In this passage, Jacob realizes the woman he is married to is not his beloved, Rachel. He is livid! Can you imagine how Leah feels to wake up to a very surprised and *very* angry Jacob? Like all of us, Leah just wants to be loved and cherished, not shamed and vulnerable. Thankfully, Jacob chooses not to confront her.

Jacob loves Rachel more than Leah. This is stated in scripture and is clear from the fact that Jacob agrees to work another seven years for Laban in order to marry Rachel a week after his marriage to Leah. Leah, used by her father to gain seven more years of labor from Jacob, is left on the sidelines. But this situation will soon change.

So far, Leah's story has described her actions rather than letting us hear from her. She is painted as quiet and going with the flow, even when things are rocky. There is wisdom in not complaining because she cannot force Jacob to love her. But she can't stay in this condition for long. We'll see internal growth as Leah learns to grab hold of what really matters. God is working behind the scenes in her life, as we will see in tomorrow's passage.

FOR REFLECTION

1. In his anger, Jacob doesn't show much regard for Leah's feelings. When you're feeling wronged, do you stop to think about who else might also have been hurt, or do you go straight to confronting the wrongdoer? Which is more important?

2. Laban denies wrongdoing and blames custom as to why he gave Leah to Jacob. Does it ever feel easier on your conscience to deceive someone by withholding information rather than telling an outright lie?

Day 3

God Gives a Blessing
Genesis 29:31

Leah's life takes a good turn, even though Jacob still does not love her and prefers her sister. She still feels the effects of being overlooked.

God sees what is going on. He sees that Jacob's feelings for Leah have not changed and blesses Leah to conceive Jacob's first child before Rachel does.

Remember that in the culture of that time, having children was an essential aspect of life. In Leah's case, this pregnancy was especially auspicious news. Through her, God will carry out the promise He made to Abraham and Isaac. This next generation of children through Jacob will start with Leah.

Leah is now looked upon with privilege and considered blessed by God for carrying the first child. She is rewarded more than Rachel and does not have to say a word about it. Remember how Sarah's servant,

Hagar, was prideful when she got pregnant? Leah may have felt that same way, but she does not boast like Hagar. Instead, she is no longer on the sidelines and can finally hold her head high.

FOR REFLECTION

1. What messages did God send Leah when he allowed her to get pregnant before Rachel? How was Leah like Hagar? How was she different? When you receive good fortune, how do you keep from becoming prideful and boasting to those who have less?

2. What does it tell us about Leah's character that she does not boast of her pregnancy to Rachel? Does boasting about something make you enjoy it more? Why do you think we're tempted to boast?

Day 4

More Than a Name
Genesis 29:32–35

During her childbearing years, Leah demonstrates "if-then" thinking: "*If* I give birth, *then* Jacob will love me." With her first son, she recognizes that God sees her misery and chooses the name Reuben, which means "son."

Leah names her second son Simeon, which means "heard." She knows God heard her prayers. She names her third son Levi, meaning "to join," indicating her hope that her husband will become attached to her at last. Leah aches, wanting some form of true connection with Jacob. She is willing to take attachment and bonding through children over love of her heart.

Leah's logic shifts with her fourth son, Judah, which means "praise." She praises God for the gifts of having children, instead of wishing for them to be a solution for her problems. She chooses to give thanks to the Creator who heard and blessed her rather than focus on Jacob's emotional abandonment. The metamorphosis is beginning in Leah's heart.

She is shifting her attention to praise and gratitude over what she lacks in love from her husband.

FOR REFLECTION

1. When Leah has Levi, she hopes that even if Jacob won't love her, he will at least become attached to her. What's the difference? Have you ever stayed connected to someone in your life even though their feelings for you weren't what you wanted? Was it a healthy decision?

2. Judah is the child whose lineage leads to Jesus. What significance do you see between Leah giving birth to Judah and the shift in her thinking? When you have been in difficult situations, what helped you shift your thinking to lead you out of the problem?

Day 5

The Metamorphosis
Genesis 30:9–21

Even though Leah praises God for her children, jealousy overtakes her when Rachel's servants bear Jacob's children because in their culture, it means these children count as Rachel's. To ease her jealousy, Leah gives her own servant to Jacob to grow her clan.

Leah gives birth to three more boys. She continues praising God rather than trying to earn Jacob's love. After she gives birth to her final son, she hopes that at the very least Jacob will honor her in some fashion for having a total of seven children with him.

Leah's self-worth has matured from hoping for crumbs of endearment from Jacob to recognizing that having children is an honorable role blessed by God. Leah softens her heart and focuses on praise. Although she is not wrong for wanting love from Jacob, she comes to realize she cannot force him to care for her.

Leah teaches us that we cannot help our feelings, but we can choose to channel our emotions into praise for what we have and not complain or impose guilt on another person because of their feelings or actions.

FOR REFLECTION

1. Have you been in situations where you had to focus your feelings on God rather than on the limitations of other people?

2. Why is Leah's transformation important?

3. Rachel thinks mandrakes will help her conceive. Has there been a time in your life when you felt you should have put more trust in God instead of chasing ineffective solutions to your problems?

Day 6

Acceptance
Genesis 30:25–43, Genesis 31:1–55

In Genesis 31, Jacob calls Leah and Rachel to talk to them about leaving their father because God has instructed Jacob to move away from Laban's land.

It is the first time we see Leah and Rachel express anger over their father's shenanigans. It is also the first time we see Jacob treat Leah as equal to Rachel, and the first time the sisters are on the same side and in agreement with each other.

Rachel steals religious idols from her father before they leave, but Leah is innocent of any wrongdoing. Leah has settled into her role as mother, with acceptance from Jacob and self-worth from God. This satisfaction culminates Leah's personal journey from a quiet woman on the sidelines to a woman with peace in her heart and a matriarch full of gratitude toward God.

1. How is Leah different in her speech about her father in this passage compared with when we first meet her? When have personal circumstances changed you?

2. Why do you think the scriptures show Rachel stealing idols and hiding them, versus Leah, who was innocent of it all? What does it tell us about Leah? What do your behaviors say about you?

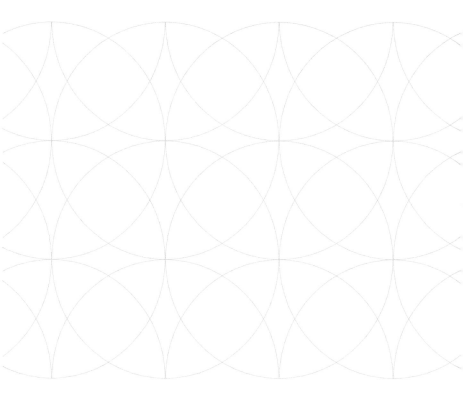

Day 7: Reflect and Take Action

KEY INSIGHTS

- Leah was used by her father to deceive Jacob, similar to how Jacob was used by his mother, Rebekah, when he deceived his father, Isaac, into giving him the blessing. It is a great example of the biblical principle of sowing and reaping (Proverbs 22:8, Galatians 6:6–10).

- Leah realizes things need to change in her life because Jacob is not showing her love after she has his children. Instead, she praises God and focuses on what she is thankful for. Leah teaches us that doing things to win praise or love from people is fruitless, but focusing on God's love can calm our hearts.

ACTION ITEMS

Leah demonstrates "if-only" thinking about herself. Such thoughts today include: If only I looked prettier, or lost weight, or had more money. If you struggle with "if-only" thinking, try focusing on what you are thankful for. Write a gratitude list in your journal as a thank-you letter to God.

Many of us can identify with Leah's feelings of being overlooked and underappreciated. What can you appreciate in yourself that others miss? Consider people in your life who may be underappreciated and show them your gratitude with words or actions.

Leah is transformed. Has your life been transformed in some way? If it has, describe these changes in your journal. If not, how would you like it to change? Make a list of items you'll need for this change. Start with a change in your thinking, like Leah did.

RAHAB: AN UNCONVENTIONAL HERO

Daily Readings

Day 1: Joshua 2:1–7

Day 2: Joshua 2:8–11

Day 3: Joshua 2:12–21

Day 4: Joshua 6:1–25

Day 5: Matthew 1:5, Matthew 1:16

Day 6: James 2:24–26, Hebrews 11:31

Day 7: Reflect and Take Action

We're taking a leap in time from the story of Leah and Rachel. God changes Jacob's name to Israel in Genesis 32:22–32 as he moves his family to Egypt. About 400 years later, all of Israel's lineage are enslaved there. God chooses Moses to lead more than 600,000 Israelites to the promised land He has chosen for them.

After God leads the Israelites out of Egypt, they wander in the desert for 40 years. This is where Rahab comes into the picture. It is time for the Israelites to claim the land God promised them. Their first stop is Jericho, Rahab's city.

Rahab is an astute woman. She is a prostitute and an innkeeper, and her professions enable her to be privy to information from all over. When Joshua's spies arrive, Rahab senses that something very big is about to transpire. She has to decide quickly how to react. God chooses Rahab—a woman who is courageous, bold, savvy, trusting, and proactive—to play a key role in His plan. Her choices lead to her becoming a hero, a person of action and faith, and, many years later, kin to Jesus.

Day 1

The Turning Point
Joshua 2:1–7

Joshua, who became the leader of the Israelites upon Moses's death, sends two spies to infiltrate Jericho. They find themselves at Rahab's inn. Rahab is probably used to encountering visitors from outside Jericho. But in her conversation with the Israelites, she likely senses that God is in their words. Rather than turn the spies over to the king, she takes them to her rooftop and hides them. She knows hiding these men means risking death.

The king of Jericho learns the men are staying with Rahab and demands she turn them over. She doesn't. Instead she demonstrates great bravery and creates an elaborate plan to help these strangers who spoke of God. The Lord has chosen Rahab, an ordinary woman, to carry out His will. And Rahab's faith grows as she risks her life to be closer to the God who was growing in her heart.

FOR REFLECTION

1. As a woman who operated an inn, Rahab likely enjoyed rare independence for her time. She had a lot to lose by hiding the spies. What do you think made it worth the risk to her?

2. Rahab is a woman with humble origins. What does her becoming an unlikely hero tell us about who God calls to serve Him? Do you consider yourself to be an unlikely hero? Why?

Day 2

The Proactive Leader
Joshua 2:8-11

After Rahab sends the king's men away, she explains to the Israelites all she has learned about God.

Rahab tells the spies that she has heard about the miracles of God. She knows their God was the Creator of heaven and earth. Something in her heart tells her God is giving Jericho to the spies and their people. Based on what she has been told, she also knows her city will be destroyed so that no idols, altars to false gods, or people who worship these things will be left behind. If Rahab is terrified by this knowledge, she does not let it show.

Rahab reveals her vulnerability as she shares the fear her people have of these men and God. But we don't see her begging for her life. Instead, she acts as a leader by hiding the spies and talking with them about God.

It must have been difficult for Rahab to reach beyond her own culture and religion. But she seems to feel that something is missing or wrong, and it is her opportunity to find a new path. We can all relate to the difficulty of following our instincts when it would be easier to stick with something familiar, even when we know it isn't working for us.

FOR REFLECTION

1. In speaking with the Israelite spies, Rahab processes out loud all she knows in her heart. How does sharing her thoughts help her form a connection with the spies? Are you a conversational processer or do you keep things inside? How do you think talking to others can help you understand what is in your heart?

2. Rahab is vulnerable with the spies. Do you find it difficult or easy to be vulnerable? How do you feel when people are vulnerable with you?

Day 3

The Crimson Cord of Faith
Joshua 2:12–21

In this passage Rahab seems able to read the two spies, and so she boldly goes for what she wants.

Rahab asks them to swear on God to spare her and her family, because that oath is stronger than just asking them to save her. She understands these men hold God above everything and are unlikely to break their oath. Her faith grows in God because she puts her life on the line.

The spies negotiate by ensuring Rahab keeps silent about their plan of attack. They put into place a means to save Rahab and her family, with a crimson cord signifying where to find them. This cord and the men's oath are the only things keeping Rahab's family alive—or so she thinks. Little does she know she has been part of God's plan this whole time. Rahab's boldness, kindness, and faith are hanging from the scarlet cord in her window.

FOR REFLECTION

1. Rahab risks everything, including her family members' lives, to know the God of the spies who have come to her inn. What would you be willing to risk to achieve a closer relationship with God?

2. Rahab puts her faith in total strangers. How do you feel about trusting others, especially people you don't know? Is it difficult or easy?

| Day 4

An Honored Oath
Joshua 6:1–25

It is time for war. The inhabitants of Jericho, including Rahab and her family, must be on edge as the Israelites spend seven days marching around their city. I imagine Rahab and her whole clan constantly looking out the window, wondering what their fate will be and hoping the strangers who took the oath to save them will remember the crimson cord.

Rahab's trust is rewarded. The spies tell their leader, Joshua, all about Rahab, the courageous and faithful negotiator, and the oath they made with her. Joshua honors that oath and saves her family. Rahab and her clan are relocated outside the Israelite camp, so they do not have to witness the destruction of their city. Although Rahab's family is saved, her city is not. It is a victory for the Israelites and a complicated day for Rahab and her kin.

Rahab's life as she knows it is over. Her town, her friends, and all that was familiar no longer exist. She chooses to stay with the Israelites. Although she is thankful she and her family were spared, she will probably face difficulties living with new people and new customs. Brave and fearless Rahab has to overcome many challenges as she assimilates into her new life.

FOR REFLECTION

1. We do not hear any words spoken by Rahab in this passage. Why do you think that is? Have you ever gone through challenges you had no words for? What helped you find your words and get your footing? What brought you comfort?

2. Rahab experiences so much that day. She gives up her way of life as she knows it to save her family and follow God. Do you feel you have given up things in your life to follow Him? If so, what does it look like to you?

| Day 5

Accepted and Married
Matthew 1:5, Matthew 1:16

After the destruction of Jericho, Rahab lived with the Israelites. Although working as a prostitute is acceptable in her native culture, the Israelites do not approve. Yet she is not shunned or shamed. Her story in the book of Joshua ends there, but we learn a bit more in the book of Matthew.

The book of Matthew starts out with the genealogy of Jesus; the passages selected for today's reading highlight Rahab's place in the family tree. Most scholars claim it is the Rahab of Jericho who eventually finds love and marries Salmon, an Israelite. It is nice to know she was accepted into the Israelite clan, settled into married life, and had a happily ever after.

God chooses Rahab, our unconventional hero who initially does not worship the God of Abraham, to be an important person in Christian history. Several generations later, through Rahab and Salmon, comes Jesus. Rahab does not seem like a typical hero, but God chooses the one whose heart is willing to help, even if she does not understand the significance she will play.

FOR REFLECTION

1. Why do you think Rahab stays to live with the Israelites?

2. Rahab's movement from pagan life to worshiping God is accompanied by leaving everything behind. Is anything in your life a remnant of a time when you were less devoted to your faith? What can you let go of to move closer to God?

3. How does God's choice to use Rahab as an integral part of His plan show that her life choices in Jericho do not define who she is and that God can utilize anyone for His plans, no matter what?

Day 6

Putting Faith to Work
James 2:24–26, Hebrews 11:31

Rahab's faith and courage are discussed twice many years later, in the New Testament. The actions Rahab performs are called "works," according to James 2:24–26. She performs these works because of her faith in God. She could have sat back with the knowledge she had about God and escaped with her family. Instead, she hides the spies and sends the Jericho men on a false mission. Rahab models the idea that you need action with your faith to be righteous.

Paul, the author of Hebrews, explains that in addition to having faith in God, Rahab also welcomed the spies in peace ("friendly welcome" in the ESV translation). She is the only one who offers peace among the people of Jericho, who honor false gods and use child sacrifice in their religion. Her peace, along with her faith, saves her.

The fact that Rahab's actions are remembered well after her death is a testament to her character. She has a growing connection to God in her heart that motivates her to start with peace then move to action. Rahab is truly a model of courage, trust, leadership, and redemption.

FOR REFLECTION

1. Why is this concept of faith plus works, which Rahab demonstrates, so important? What does it look like in your own life?

2. Where do you think the peace Rahab gives to the spies comes from? How can you invite that kind of peace into your own life and also bring it to others, including strangers?

Day 7: Reflect and Take Action

KEY INSIGHTS

- Rahab illustrates her courage by risking death if she is found out. Her bravery and quick decisions seem rooted in her desire to grow closer to God, whom she has heard of but knows little about. Today it's much easier for us to learn about God, but are we willing to make even minor sacrifices to grow closer to Him?

- Rahab solves problems and improvises in her story, creating a swift plan to hide the spies and throw off the Jericho men. She is smart and quick-thinking.

- Rahab's story gives us a beautiful picture of redemption, as her desire to know God saves her from unspeakable horror and the corruption of her own culture's religion, and guides her to become one of God's people.

ACTION ITEMS

How does Rahab's story model the importance of acceptance? Do you accept others? Why or why not? Ask God to help you see others through His eyes to be more accepting, and be intentional this week (and beyond) to be accepting of other people.

Many people have experienced trauma in their lives. If you have, consider seeking help to release it. Start looking for your special helper this week. You can start by looking for a referral from your local church or cathedral, Therapyforchristians.com, or PsychologyToday.com.

Rahab isn't afraid, even though she is in a dangerous situation. Most of us experience fear occasionally. Read Psalm 46:1–3 and Psalm 23:4. How can these verses help you the next time you are afraid? Record your thoughts in your journal.

DEBORAH: A POWERFUL VOICE IN A TIME OF WAR

Daily Readings

Day 1: Judges 4:1–5

Day 2: Judges 4:6–8

Day 3: Judges 4:9–10, Romans 15:1–2

Day 4: Judges 4:12–24

Day 5: Judges 5:1–7

Day 6: Judges 5:8–31

Day 7: Reflect and Take Action

Deborah is quite the woman. The only female judge mentioned in the Bible, she is also a prophet, poet, and leader who is forthright and encouraging with her people. Before we meet Deborah, we learn the Jewish people rebelled against God after the last prophet, Ehud, died. Because of this revolt, God allows them to be given to their enemy, the Canaanites. King Jabin's army leader, Sisera, cruelly oppresses the Israelites for 20 years before they cry out to God for help.

This is when we meet Deborah, sitting under a palm tree about 13 miles outside Jerusalem, judging matters for the Israelites. In those days, judges not only settled disputes but could also be military commanders.

A prophet of strength, faith, and encouragement, Deborah helps lead the Israelite army through her encouragement of Barak, God's chosen commander. Her straightforward prophecy and wisdom serve her people greatly while keeping their focus on God. Deborah even shows her artistic side by singing poetry and praises to the Lord for the great victory He brought about. Because of Deborah, and her powerful voice, the Israelites live in peace for 40 more years.

Day 1

Deborah's Palm Tree
Judges 4:1–5

In Judges 3 we learn the Israelites go in and out of their relationship with God. Because they live with and marry the Canaanites, they are influenced by the culture and began to worship their spouses' gods. They then become oppressed by an enemy ruler and cry out to God for relief.

After the death of Ehud, Deborah is chosen to be the next prophet, and only female judge, for Israel. In those days, a judge dealt with matters within the Israelite society, but they could also lead their military, as Ehud did. A prophet is a spokesperson for God. We first meet Deborah, the wise servant, presiding as a judge for her people, settling disputes under a palm tree named after her.

Men usually held Deborah's job. The fact that the Israelites seek her help shows that they regard her as wise and benevolent. She teaches us that doing your job well garners respect, which isn't limited by gender.

FOR REFLECTION

1. Sometimes our job overlaps or translates nicely into a different one. How do you think judging matters for the Israelites could

help Deborah be a strong military leader? Can you think of a time when something you learned in one context—whether a job skill, a classroom lesson, or another experience—turned out to be helpful in a different situation?

2. What traits does Deborah demonstrate that draw the Israelites to her for judgment? Who in your life has similar traits? Have you complimented them on these characteristics?

Day 2

The Encourager
Judges 4:6-8

Deborah sends for Barak and reminds him what God commanded him to do. (She must have told him before because she is refreshing his memory.) Barak tells Deborah he will go to war only if she goes with him.

Barak is not motivated or willing to go to war on his own. But Deborah intervenes and tells him what she knows to hold him accountable. She encourages Barak by reminding him that God promised that he would be the one to take out their oppressor. Yet Barak has little faith.

Deborah, however, has strong faith. She heard God's message and relayed it without fear. She even spells out her role of bringing victory to Barak. We can see Barak struggle to take on his role. Accepting what God asks of us is not always easy. When you struggle in this way, do you seek people like Deborah who will encourage you with their strong faith?

FOR REFLECTION

1. Why do you think Deborah calls for Barak when she does? Can you think of a time when you had to remind someone of their duty? Do you think you handled it in the best way? What about a time when you were the hesitant one?

2. Barak asks Deborah to go to war with him. Why do you think he does so? Would things have been different if he had simply asked her without refusing to go otherwise? Do you find it easy or difficult to ask someone to support you through a difficult undertaking?

Day 3

The Ultimatum
Judges 4:9–10, Romans 15:1–2

In yesterday's reading we learned Barak tried to make a deal with God, stating he would do God's will only if Deborah went with him. He gives Deborah an ultimatum, threatening to abandon his duty if he doesn't get his way. Deborah knows the importance of this war and has no fear because God is with the Israelites. Because of Barak's choice, she tells him directly that he will now have to go to war without personal victory. A woman will take Sisera out instead and get the glory meant for Barak.

Deborah does not coddle Barak. She is direct and tells Barak what God told her. We witness her obedience, strong faith, and her bravery. Deborah is a commanding woman who does not beat around the bush.

Isn't it interesting that a woman is given the honor that Barak passes up, a role typically played by a male hero? As with Deborah herself, this outcome is a reminder that God's decisions are not limited by our typical gender stereotypes. It should give us pause when making assumptions of what someone is capable of based on their gender. God can put anyone into His plans, even if it seems unconventional.

FOR REFLECTION

1. Deborah tells Barak, "The road on which you are going will not lead to your glory." Do you sometimes need a reminder that you are on the wrong path for your life? Who do you trust to give you that feedback?

2. How does Romans 15:1–2 apply to Deborah and what she did for Barak? Do you ever find it difficult to bear with someone else's weaknesses? Can you think of a time when someone encouraged you when you didn't have the strength you needed?

Day 4

Into a Woman's Hands
Judges 4:12-24

A few days later, God tells Deborah the day for battle is here. To offer hope, Deborah reminds Barak that God is ahead and has put things in order.

They go to battle with only swords against Sisera and his 900 iron chariots. The Israelites are at a disadvantage. But God confuses and destroys the enemy. Sisera's whole army is killed by the Israelites. Sisera himself runs away into the tent of a woman named Jael. Little does he know Jael is the woman who Deborah prophesied would kill him.

Deborah is a courageous and powerful leader to her people while also giving hope and encouragement to Barak, getting him to follow through with commanding the Israelites to war. Being a great leader like Deborah includes inspiring others as well as giving commands. Deborah knows she is not to take Barak's role and that he has his part to play.

FOR REFLECTION

1. We see Deborah give hope to Barak after she tells him to get up and go. Why does she do so, as opposed to simply commanding him as a judge and prophet? What is the lesson?

2. Deborah can be authoritative, too. Why do you think she needs to be tough with Barak and not rely solely on inspiring him with hope? Can you think of times in your life when you needed to both motivate someone and be strict with them? How do you balance those two methods?

Day 5

A Mother to Israel
Judges 5:1–7

The war is won, and Sisera is dead. Barak has fulfilled his role, as has Deborah. It is now time to celebrate by praising God in a poem and singing, interweaving the story of the war. Deborah and Barak sing this song as equals. She honors and respects the role Barak has played and treats him accordingly.

Deborah gives honor and praise to God for all He has done. She praises all the men who helped win the war and even gives herself a pat on the back. As a mother to her people, Deborah demonstrates that when God works in your life, it's important to acknowledge and thank Him, as well as everyone who stepped up to help.

Deborah's treatment of Barak is also notable. She is wise and generous to include him in her song and not dwell on his flaws. As a judge, Deborah shows that judgment can include mercy and understanding— which we all need, because none of us are perfect.

FOR REFLECTION

1. Deborah expresses her devotion and emotions in an artful manner by using poetry and song. How do you express your gratitude to God or others? Do you ever get creative?

2. Consider the many roles Deborah plays in this story—judge, leader, prophet, inspirer. How have you played these roles in your life? How have you honored God in these roles?

Day 6

Deborah Paints a Picture
Judges 5:8–31

Deborah continues to sing. Her song explains when the floods came and filled the river of Kishon, the river was the water that took out Sisera and his men. She honors Jael for slaying Sisera. (We don't know if Jael is a sympathizer or an Israelite, nor do we know her motivation.)

Deborah then sings about Sisera's mother, wondering if her son and his men would take women as spoils. Instead, Jael took Sisera captive. Deborah ends her song cursing the enemy and blessing God's friends.

This song serves many purposes. Deborah is proud of her people and lifts up all those who participated in God's plan of war by thanking them. She also reminds everyone it was God's strength, not theirs, that made this victory possible. She refers to the consequences of war by mentioning those who have fallen and their families, like Sisera and his mother. She reminds listeners of the reason for the conflict, which is the suffering of the Israelites under Sisera.

FOR REFLECTION

1. Why do you think Deborah sings about the days leading up to the war, as well as the details of the war itself? How do you confront difficult news?

2. Singing praises to God is a common theme throughout the Bible; in fact, "psalms" actually means "songs." Miriam, Moses's sister, is the first woman to sing praises to God, in Exodus 15:21. The Sons of Korah wrote Psalm 47, and King David wrote Psalm 108, both of which were created after Deborah wrote her song, and both give praise to God. How is Deborah's song the same as the songs in those readings? How are they different? What are they like compared with modern-day praise songs?

Day 7: Reflect and Take Action

KEY INSIGHTS

- Deborah is a prophet and the only female judge named in the Bible. Her role is surprising because men usually handled war. She reminds us God can choose anyone to use as His instrument.

- Deborah is forthright and faithful to God. She tells it like it is and doesn't worry about what Barak thinks of her or his fear of war. There is no people-pleasing with Deborah.

- Deborah helps Barak come into his calling as a commander by treating him as one and calls him a leader in her song. She doesn't condemn him for his flaws or act superior because she has greater faith. She tries to bring out the best in him.

ACTION ITEMS

It can be easy to be critical of people and can be challenging to encourage them. Deborah encouraged. Search what the Bible says about encouragement. Then encourage people in your life this week (and beyond) and notice how they respond to you.

Here is your chance to get creative: Write a poem or song of praise to God for something in your life. Take notice if there were other people involved and include them. Write it in your notebook or journal.

Deborah sang about Sisera's mother. How do you think others paint a picture of you? Ask your family and friends their thoughts. Is that how you want to be remembered? If not, what needs to change? How can you start to make those changes?

RUTH: THE REDEEMED

Daily Readings

Day 1: Ruth 1:1–22

Day 2: Ruth 2:1–17

Day 3: Ruth 2:18–23

Day 4: Ruth 3:1–10

Day 5: Ruth 3:11–18

Day 6: Ruth 4:1–17

Day 7: Reflect and Take Action

We enter this chapter in 1140 BC, about 95 years after Deborah and Barak go to war. Ruth, a recent widow, chooses to follow her mother-in-law, Naomi, to an unfamiliar city and culture, much like Rahab did when she joined the Israelites.

Redemption is the theme of Ruth's story. Boaz is literally called her redeemer because when a woman was widowed, the closest single male relative had the option to marry her and ensure she was taken care of.

During Ruth's story, we learn she is devoted, strong, loving, determined, humble, gentle, kind, and obedient—all during times of great stress, personal hardship, and sadness. Her union with Boaz takes place in Bethlehem, the future birthplace of their descendent Jesus, who is the Redeemer for us all.

Ruth is blameless for being a widow and poor. She is a victim of circumstance, trying to do what she can under the customs of the day. Her difficulties do not cause her to abandon Naomi, and she never gives up. She teaches us that despite our circumstances, we can rise up by being kind, helping others by working hard, asking for help when we need it, and trusting that God watches over us.

Day 1

Ruth Follows Naomi
Ruth 1:1–22

Before we meet Ruth, we meet her mother-in-law, Naomi. With her husband, Elimelech, Naomi and their two sons moved from Bethlehem to Moab. Naomi's sons married Ruth and Orpah, both of whom were Moabites.

Naomi's husband and her two sons die, leaving her sad and bitter with immeasurable grief. Because of lack of food in Moab, Naomi is motivated to return to her hometown of Bethlehem, a 50-mile trek. Although Orpah stays with her clan in Moab, Ruth chooses to go with Naomi.

Ruth chooses to care for Naomi even though Naomi is grieving and is not easy to be around. She chooses the difficult path of leaving her country and becoming a foreigner in an unfamiliar city. In addition, Ruth tells Naomi she chooses to worship Naomi's God. Perhaps witnessing how Naomi's family made God a priority in their home touches Ruth's heart, inspiring her to make this life-altering decision.

After choosing to follow God, Ruth immediately puts her faith into practice by staying with Naomi in her time of need. Ruth teaches us to be kind to those who are hurting and to be women of our word.

1. Do you think Naomi's struggles have anything to do with Ruth choosing to stay with her? Why or why not? Has anyone ever stood by you during an especially difficult time, even though they weren't obligated? How did it feel?

2. What characteristics does Ruth demonstrate in this passage? Does she remind you of anyone you know?

Day 2

Hope Fulfilled
Ruth 2:1–17

Poor and hungry, Ruth and Naomi make it to Bethlehem. Ruth's only option for survival is picking leftover grain in the fields. She ends up in a field belonging to a man named Boaz (who is related to Rahab), who is from the clan of Elimelech, Naomi's late husband. Ruth's hope of being noticed by a kind man is fulfilled. Boaz makes sure she gets extra grain, feeds her, and ensures she stays on his land to protect her.

Ruth wonders how Boaz could be so kind to her given that she is not from Bethlehem. He explains he has already heard about her kindness to Naomi and wants to repay her. The assistance Ruth has been longing for has arrived, as well as the beginning of a romance.

Ruth and Naomi are at a very low point in their lives, even though they are together. God intervenes, leading Ruth to Boaz, who recognizes the selflessness she has shown to his kinswoman. Ruth's story demonstrates that God takes notice of us in our troubles and brings people into our lives when we are in need.

FOR REFLECTION

1. Is it easy or difficult for you to help strangers? What do you think about others who are struggling, especially those whom you do not know personally?

2. How is helping the poor in Ruth's time the same as how we support the poor today? How is it different?

Day 3

Redeemer Revealed
Ruth 2:18–23

Seeing all the grain Ruth brings home, Naomi wants to know more about her day. After Ruth shares, she learns her protector, Boaz, can act as a redeemer for them because he is in Naomi's family.

Gleaning the fields is dangerous for women. Ruth is brave to work there and wise to listen to the warnings. Ruth allows Boaz to protect her by staying with the other women on his land.

As we witness the closeness of Naomi and Ruth, we see the importance of deep relationships in helping us get through hard times. Each has different strengths: Ruth is able to gather food, and Naomi is able to teach her about staying safe. Ruth's story reminds us to appreciate our friendships and notice the strengths we bring to each other.

FOR REFLECTION

1. When Ruth carries home the heavy load of grain without complaint, what does it tell us about her character? What keeps you persevering and working hard during difficult times?

2. Because Ruth married one of Naomi's sons, she is part of the family even after his death. Do you think being a daughter-in-law today means being part of a family on the same level Ruth is to Naomi? How is it the same? How is it different?

3. How does your definition of family go beyond blood relations? Who in your life do you consider part of your family even though you're not related? Does that person know you consider them family?

Day 4

An Unusual Proposal
Ruth 3:1–10

Naomi, understanding how hard Ruth is working, wants to give Ruth a break. But the only solution she can see is for Ruth to marry so she will no longer need to gather grain in the field all day. Naomi gives Ruth specific instructions on how to let Boaz know she honors and respects him and wants him to be her husband. These instructions may sound strange to us, but it was the way things were done in Naomi's culture at the time. Ruth does not question Naomi's advice.

Ruth follows Naomi's directions by lying at Boaz's feet while he is at the threshing floor, making it clear that she wants him to marry her as her redeemer. Boaz knows exactly what she is doing and is grateful Ruth has chosen him. Ruth appeals to Boaz's compassion as a way to escape the strict confines of her culture. Even with customs that seem strange or strict, compassion is a universal virtue we can recognize and offer to everyone.

FOR REFLECTION

1. Naomi gives Ruth very specific instructions about how to let Boaz know she wants to marry him. What do you think lying at Boaz's feet represents? How do you get what you need or want from someone?

2. Ruth has to swallow all her pride and plead for help. Does your pride ever prevent you from admitting you need help? How do you get past it?

Day 5

Ruth's Worthiness
Ruth 3:11–18

In this passage, Boaz tells Ruth that all who know her think she is a worthy woman, and although he is willing to be her redeemer, there is a potential obstacle. By law, a closer relative to Ruth's late husband has the right of first refusal.

We can clearly see the strong feelings Ruth and Boaz have for each other. Although women were not allowed on the threshing floor, Boaz wants her to stay with him. In the morning Boaz does not want anyone to know she is there because she is a single woman and this knowledge could ruin her reputation (and his). Ruth, known for her worthy character, shows her boldness again, just like when she left her home in Moab with Naomi. Being redeemed appears to be more than just an agreement between the two of them and worth taking a risk. It's apparent that Boaz and Ruth care about each other and that Ruth will be redeemed out of love.

Taking a chance and being bold is something we can all aspire to. Ruth, who is humble, demonstrates it with grace. She does not second-guess Naomi but instead perseveres to get what she needs, being honest in her feelings and her actions.

FOR REFLECTION

1. Why do you think Naomi sends Ruth to the threshing floor, given that women are not allowed there? Have you ever had to take a risk or break a rule to gain attention or prove your determination? What was the result?

2. Ruth makes a bold move with an act that is not typical of women at the time, but she does so with grace. What would being bold with grace look like in your own life?

Day 6

The Marriage of Ruth and Boaz
Ruth 4:1–17

The tension raised in our last reading is resolved as Boaz offers the other family redeemer a chance to purchase Naomi's property and become the husband of Ruth, fulfilling her deceased husband's role. The kinsman turns it down, and Boaz publicly declares he will be Naomi and Ruth's redeemer. The elders give Boaz a blessing that Ruth will be like Leah and Rachel (Jacob's wives, whom we read about in week 3) in honor of Naomi's deceased husband and son.

After Ruth and Boaz are married, she conceives quickly. Naomi's friends are thrilled because she now has cause to be joyful after so much loss, sadness, and bitterness. She is no longer in poverty and has a grandchild, Obed (whose name means "service"). Ruth continues to bless Naomi by allowing her to be Obed's nurse, or caretaker.

It is moving that Ruth's success and happiness is also Naomi's success and happiness. Ruth teaches us that choosing to stand by our word with people can lead to family-like bonds.

FOR REFLECTION

1. Boaz brings the elders of Bethlehem to the meeting he has with the other family redeemer. Why do you think it is important for Boaz to have them there? At what important events in your life would you want friends, family, and the community to be witnesses?

2. How do you think Ruth's son, Obed, helped Naomi find joy again and move forward? Did something in your life bring you joy when you were feeling particularly down and defeated?

Day 7: Reflect and Take Action

KEY INSIGHTS

- Ruth insists on taking care of Naomi until death. Ruth is determined and loyal. Do you have friends who are similar to Ruth? Are you loyal and kind to your friends?

- Ruth does not realize Boaz will be her redeemer when she first meets him on his field. More than 1,000 years later, on or near this field, an angel appears to shepherds to announce Jesus, the Son of God and our Redeemer, has been born. Redemption is not just a theme for Ruth; it becomes real for all Christians.

- Ruth shows us how important it is to keep our word. She promises to care for Naomi and does so even after marriage. How important is it to you to follow through on a promise?

ACTION ITEMS

Helping those in need can look different for each of us. Have you considered what it means to you? Search for local philanthropic organizations to find a way to help. Consider donating your time, goods, or experience instead of money. Plan on following through to help those in need.

We see Ruth as fit and strong. How important are fitness and strength to you? Try adding some exercise to your routine this week to see how you feel.

ESTHER: THE COURAGEOUS YOUNG QUEEN

Daily Readings

Day 1: Esther 2:2–18

Day 2: Esther 2:19–23, Esther 3:1–15, Esther 4:1–17

Day 3: Esther 5:1–8

Day 4: Esther 5:9–14, Esther 6:1–13

Day 5: Esther 6:14, Esther 7:1–10

Day 6: Esther 8:1–17, Esther 9:1–32

Day 7: Reflect and Take Action

Esther's story occurs about 660 years after Ruth marries Boaz. (By the way, Esther and Ruth are the only two books of the Bible titled with female names.) Although God is not explicitly mentioned in this story, His favor is all over it.

Queen Esther was not always a queen; she grows up as a beautiful Jewish girl with no intentions of royalty. In an ancient beauty pageant of sorts, she is picked to win King Ahasuerus's (pronounced

"A-hash-ver-ros") favor to be his new wife. This king is not an Israelite, and Esther's uncle Mordecai (pronounced "More-de-kye") instructs her not to tell the king of her heritage, at least not in the beginning of her story.

A plot begins when King Ahasuerus's servant, Haman, wants to annihilate the Jewish people. Queen Esther devises a bold, courageous plan to stop and overturn the threat.

Esther is described as young and pretty, but we can see from her story that she is much more. God chooses her to take the role of queen. She is humble, brave, heroic, smart, and caring. Queen Esther saves her people by fasting, relying on God's wisdom, and showing courage. A rare example in the scriptures of a woman holding worldly authority, Queen Esther is much like Deborah, whom we met in week 5 of our study: wise and thoughtful in how she exercises her influence.

Day 1

From Esther to Queen
Esther 2:2–18

In today's passage, Persian King Ahasuerus desires a new wife, and Esther is in the running. She is pretty and catches the king's attention, but her uncle Mordecai warns her not to share her Jewish heritage.

As part of the king's harem, Esther is given many luxuries, including cosmetics and servants, that she would not have otherwise had. But she listens to the advice of the eunuch in charge and never takes more than she needs to the king's palace. People notice and like her.

After all the preparations, King Ahasuerus chooses humble and gracious Esther to be his wife. He places the crown on her head, holds a massive feast in her honor, and offers generous gifts. Esther, the fetching Jewish girl, is now Queen Esther, whose husband rules from India to Ethiopia.

God looks into the hearts of people (1 Samuel 16:7), and He chooses Esther to be queen at least partly because of her humility. Being humble does not mean being weak, as we will learn from Esther and her journey of triumph.

1. Why do you think Mordecai warns Esther not to share her heritage? Are you ever tempted to keep parts of yourself secret from other people? Is it something you want to do, or do you feel you have to?

2. Esther listens to the eunuch's advice and takes only what she needs to the palace. Why do you think this wins her favor? In your own life, do you think material possessions (or lack of) affect people's perceptions of you? Is it a good thing?

| Day 2

Esther's Courage Grows
Esther 2:19–23, Esther 3:1–15, Esther 4:1–17

After Esther is chosen to marry King Ahasuerus, Mordecai overhears two people threatening to kill the king. He tells Esther, she warns the king, and the threat is eliminated. Mordecai's warning is recorded in the royal chronicles, which is important a bit later in our study.

Danger arises as King Ahasuerus appoints Haman to a position in which people have to bow to him. Mordecai does not bow because he is Jewish. This defiance infuriates Haman. He decides to kill Mordecai and the Jewish people because they won't bow to him. When the royal decree is sent throughout the kingdom, Mordecai sends word and begs Queen Esther to save her people by going to the king. Initially, she declines and makes excuses, showing herself to be human with doubts and fears. But Mordecai explains that she may have been granted her position as queen so she can help her people in their time of need. She commands her people to fast as her courage grows.

1. Queen Esther asks all her people to fast on her behalf as a way for her to become open to God's plan for protection. How do you handle challenging or hazardous situations? Do you pray? Fast? Ask others to do the same?

2. At what point does Queen Esther change her mind about talking to the king? When have you felt your courage grow and taken a different course of action?

3. Considering that God had a purpose for making her queen seemed to give Esther courage. How often do you consider that God may have given you blessings so you can do good works?

Day 3

The Fasting Plan
Esther 5:1–8

After three days of fasting, it is apparent that God puts a plan in Queen Esther's heart to save her people from annihilation. She dresses in her royal robes and stands outside the king's throne room to get his attention. He sees her, agrees to hear her, and offers her whatever she wants. Instead of asking him to change the decree that would kill her people, Esther invites the king and Haman to a feast.

At this feast, the king asks Esther her wishes and states he is willing to give her anything she desires. She still holds back and offers another feast the next day. Her plan is unfolding.

Esther likely knows a direct appeal to the king will fail. The stakes couldn't have been higher, but she keeps her cool. Instead of openly demanding the king change his mind, Queen Esther is gracious and kind, offering a feast in his honor. She holds back her anger and emotions, working carefully to expose Haman's true nature.

1. Why do you think Queen Esther holds back her request and instead offers a feast to the king? Have you ever found that directly demanding what you wanted just made things worse?

2. Queen Esther's plan includes Haman. She not only understands what the king needs, but also knows how Haman's mind works. How well do you understand the needs of people in your life?

Day 4

Behind the Scenes Queen
Esther 5:9–14, Esther 6:1–13

An interesting parallel takes place in this passage. On the same night Haman makes his plan to hang Mordecai, a sleepless King Ahasuerus hears from the royal book of chronicles that Mordecai was never honored for saving his life.

This revelation sets up the comeuppance for Haman the next day. He assumes the king wants to honor him, only to find out that Mordecai will receive the elaborate treatment that Haman suggested. Haman's plan to kill Mordecai is rendered futile, and instead he has to grant Mordecai the celebration he has inadvertently designed.

Although God isn't directly mentioned in today's passage, His influence is clear. The king becomes aware of his debt to Mordecai at exactly the right moment to spare his life. It is apparent that God put Esther in her role, where the quiet queen can work behind the scenes to turn the fate of her people.

FOR REFLECTION

1. What are the signs that God has put Queen Esther in her royal position? What events are likely unfolding without her? Can you think of a time in your own life when you seemed to be in just the right place and situation to help someone or do a good deed?

2. Everything that played out in this section could be looked at as coincidence if you fail to consider God's involvement. What have you seen in your own life that looked like a coincidence but had to be God?

Day 5

The Plan Is in Motion
Esther 6:14, Esther 7:1–10

At the second feast, it becomes clear that Esther was wise to proceed as she had. After the king is reminded that his life was spared and enjoys two planned feasts in his honor, Queen Esther asks if he is pleased with her. What could he say but yes? Now the moment is right, and Esther asks the king to spare her life and those of her people.

Queen Esther keeps her composure during the feast, and even when the king asks about her request, she remains humble. Only when she sees the king is upset about the plot against the Israelites does she finally get angry, calling out Haman as a wicked enemy. Notice that Queen Esther does not get angry at the king; she does not point out that he approved the annihilation or try to make him feel guilty. Instead, she focuses on Haman. We learn from the Esther to focus on the injustice at hand, get to the root of it, and allow the people unknowingly involved to feel the weight of their guilt and make a change. And the king does just that.

FOR REFLECTION

1. How do you think Queen Esther kept her composure during the feast before she called out Haman? Do you keep your composure during times of distress? If so, how? If not, what could you do differently?

2. Esther does not deceive the king, but she is strategic about when and how she reveals things to him. Do you see a difference? Does what's at stake affect the correctness of her approach?

3. Queen Esther does not use guilt as a motivator for change with the king. How do you persuade people to see things from your perspective or make important changes?

Day 6

Coming of Age
Esther 8:1–17, Esther 9:1–32

After Haman is killed, King Ahasuerus gives Mordecai Haman's job. But the danger has not passed. Queen Esther pleads with the king to reverse the edict, but the king's signet ring on a decree means it cannot be overturned. The king allows Mordecai to draft new legislation, however, which allows the Jewish people to fight back when the armies come after them. The Israelites are able to catch their enemies by surprise and defeat them.

Queen Esther, although young and humble, becomes fearless as she stands up for her people. She shows us a different kind of leader. She is a queen of human nature who trusts God for His protection, knows how to appeal to the king's emotions, and creates a yearly commemoration of an important victory called Purim that is still celebrated today.

FOR REFLECTION

1. Why is it important for Queen Esther and Mordecai to create Purim as a memorial of these events? Have you created memorials for certain events in your own life? What were they about, and what did you do to commemorate them?

2. Queen Esther is destined to become a leader, regardless of whether she wants to. Do you like being a leader, or do you prefer to be led?

3. How does Queen Esther show strength in leadership? How do you show strength in leadership in certain roles of your life?

Day 7: Reflect and Take Action

KEY INSIGHTS

- Esther knows the importance of fasting. It can help people hear God better, mourn, and purify, and it can be a ritual to gain God's favor. In this case, it is apparent that God gives her a plan that saves her people.

- Queen Esther exemplifies courage by wearing her royal robes while going into the king's quarters. The robes displayed confidence in her role as queen. Do you notice a difference in your demeanor based on the clothes you wear?

- Esther is gracious and kind. She is kind to the king even after she learns he had agreed to the edict against her people. Is it hard for you to be kind to people when you know they have wronged you?

ACTION ITEMS

Esther demonstrates respect for her uncle, the king, and others. What does respect mean to you? How do you show it? Try being more mindful of respect toward yourself, God, and others this week and beyond.

Fasting is the pivotal point for Queen Esther to hear God's plan and gather her courage. Try fasting for a day or two this week in response to an issue in your life. If it is not an option because of medical concerns or for other reasons, fast from something like social media or another activity you enjoy. Pray about your issue while fasting and ask God for His wisdom.

MARY: THE HUMBLE MOTHER OF JESUS

Daily Readings

Day 1: Luke 1:26–38

Day 2: Matthew 1:18–25, Luke 1:5–25, Luke 1:39–56

Day 3: Luke 2:1–7

Day 4: Luke 2:8–21

Day 5: Luke 2:22–52

Day 6: John 2:1–11, John 19:25–27

Day 7: Reflect and Take Action

Scattered throughout the Old Testament are prophecies about a Son being born to a virgin (Isaiah 7:14). This Son will change everything. Mary, a humble, poor, betrothed young woman, is chosen to be the mother to Jesus, the prophesied Son. She reacts with humility and sensibility. When Mary gives birth to Jesus, other people prophesy over him. She holds these words in her heart. She does not tell the world about Jesus; instead, she listens and observes.

We witness her raising Jesus as a humble mother with a quiet spirit. She is not prideful despite Jesus being the Son of God.

We learn that Mary keeps silent about her big and important news about Jesus. We see her obedience and practicality as she realizes she has a very special job to carry out. Mary demonstrates the qualities God sees in her heart that make her the chosen one, mother of the Lord of all.

| Day 1

Mary Agrees
Luke 1:26–38

Before Jesus's birth, Mary is betrothed to Joseph, which is stronger than an engagement. Back then, if you were betrothed and you cheated on your intended, you could be killed. The angel Gabriel tells Mary she will become pregnant before she is married. This news could have been a death sentence, but Mary does not take it as such.

After Gabriel informs Mary she has been chosen to carry Jesus, he explains that Elizabeth, her older relative, is also pregnant and says, "For nothing will be impossible for God." Sound familiar? Remember when Sarah laughed when she overheard she would be pregnant at age 90? It seemed impossible, but not for God. This passage depicts a parallel situation: God will put Jesus into Mary's womb, yet Mary will remain a virgin, something only God can make possible.

Gabriel tells Mary that God has found favor with her. Mary is surprised not by the angel but rather the message. She is not prideful but instead wonders why she is greeted in this way. Gabriel goes on to explain the experience that lies ahead of her. Instead of panicking that she will be pregnant before marriage, Mary has a practical response. Trusting in God, she agrees.

1. When Gabriel visits Mary, why do you think she is not surprised to see an angel but more concerned about his message? How would you feel if you encountered an angel?

2. What does Mary's final response to Gabriel reveal about her character and what she was capable of? Have you ever felt that God called you to do something difficult or unexpected or that you weren't sure you could do? How did you handle it? How hard is it for you to put your trust in God when life throws you unexpected curves?

Day 2

Mother of My Lord
Matthew 1:18–25, Luke 1:5–25, Luke 1:39–56

Joseph is also visited by the angel Gabriel, who explains what is happening to Mary. He instructs Joseph to still marry her. Joseph does so but does not consummate the marriage until after Jesus is born.

While she is pregnant, Mary visits Elizabeth, whom God has also blessed with pregnancy. Gabriel tells Elizabeth's husband, Zacharias, that his wife will conceive a son who will "make ready for the Lord a people prepared." Zacharias doubts and is made mute until their son is born.

By visiting Elizabeth, Mary confirms they have both experienced miracles. Mary sings a song of praise to God. We learn from Mary the importance of focusing not on the miracles themselves but on God, who blesses the humble and takes care of His people.

FOR REFLECTION

1. How often do you find yourself feeling doubts about God's plan for you, as opposed to trusting in Him? Do you think most people have doubts at some point?

2. How does Elizabeth know that Mary is "the mother of my Lord"? Do you think spending time together helps both Mary and Elizabeth handle their respective situations? Can you think of a time when you were able to support someone even as they supported you?

3. Why is Mary's song important to her story? What does it say about her? Is her song similar to Deborah's from week 5? Why or why not?

Day 3

Mary Doesn't Complain
Luke 2:1–7

As Joseph and Mary travel to Bethlehem, Mary is still described as Joseph's betrothed. Experts say they must have had a wedding, but because they have not been intimate (see Matthew 1:25), they are not yet fully married. In ancient Hebrew culture, marriage was not official until it was consummated.

Mary and Joseph are turned away from all the inns and cannot find a place to stay. There are a couple of theories as to where Mary gives birth: either in a barn or in a home that shared space with farm animals. Regardless, Mary gives birth to Jesus in humble surroundings, swaddles Him in a blanket, and places Him in a feeding trough called a manger.

We do not see Mary complain about walking around 90 miles to Bethlehem while being very pregnant or about sharing her birthing spot with animals. Most of all, she does not question why she has to place her son in a feeding trough when He would have the throne of David. Mary is patient, calm, and good-natured in these arduous circumstances. She is steadfast with her trust in God's plan.

1. Why is it important that the scriptures tell us that Mary was still betrothed to Joseph? What does it tell us about Mary and the prophecies?

2. Mary's patience with her circumstances reminds us a bit of Ruth, from week 6 of our study. How is Mary similar to Ruth, and how is she different? What lessons can you take from each of them?

3. Why do you think Mary does not question God and the conditions in which Jesus is brought into the world? What do you do when it's hard to see how your current situation will lead to the outcome you expect or want?

| Day 4

Pondering in Her Heart
Luke 2:8–21

Shepherds are tending sheep at night near the field where we met Ruth and Boaz (from week 6). Suddenly an angel and God's glory appear. The angel tells the shepherds about the birth of Jesus and how He was sent from God to be the Messiah. After the shepherds find Jesus, they tell many people about the things they have seen. They also tell Mary and Joseph what the angel has told them. Mary does not say anything but instead "treasured up all these things, pondering them in her heart."

After eight days, Jesus is circumcised and given His name. Remember that His name was given before He was conceived. Mary is compliant with giving him this name, which means "Jehovah is salvation." She is adding all she heard from Gabriel to the shepherds' stories about her precious son. Mary is quiet, but knowledge is building inside her soul. Mary shows us the value of making time to contemplate God's work in our lives and words spoken by others that praise God's Word. It is a great reminder to ponder God's Word in our hearts.

1. Why do you think it is important for the scriptures to remind us that Jesus's name was given before He was conceived?

2. What does it say about Mary that she treasures up all these things and ponders them? How can you follow this example in your own life?

Day 5

Mary Remains Humble
Luke 2:22–52

When Simeon prophesies over Jesus, He reveals that Jesus will be a light to the Gentiles and glory for the Israelites. He also says Mary's soul will be pierced. Mary and Joseph marvel at this news.

When Jesus is 12, His family travels to Jerusalem for Passover. When it is time to leave, Jesus stays behind without his parents' knowledge. When they finally find Him three days later, Jesus explains that He had to be in His Father's house. In this moment, Mary does not understand what Jesus means.

Mary doesn't believe she has special privilege because she was chosen to give birth to Jesus. Instead, she follows the laws and customs of her day. She takes in all that Simeon prophesies. She adds Jesus's words at the temple to what is already in her heart.

Mary is a model of motherhood. She watches Jesus mature, is surprised by Him, listens to Him, and fears for His safety. Any parent can relate to these experiences. Although Jesus is the most important child to be born on earth, we can learn from Mary how to honor the unique qualities in all our children today by listening and supporting them.

FOR REFLECTION

1. Mary is chosen by God to carry His only Son, but she never uses this distinction to her advantage. Mary is mindful of her privilege

and models humility. What are some privileges you have? How can you follow Mary's example and set them aside?

2. Why do you think Mary does not understand what Jesus means when He says he had to be in His Father's house? Have you ever misunderstood someone when they said something important? When did you learn you were wrong? Did you resolve it? Why or why not?

Day 6

Mary Encourages Jesus
John 2:1–11, John 19:25–27

Jesus starts his teaching ministry around 19 years after we leave Mary in Jerusalem at Passover. One day Jesus, His disciples, and Mary attend a wedding in Cana. Back then, weddings were held over several days. It was the wedding party's responsibility to provide food and drink for the duration of the celebration. If they ran out, it brought great shame to the family.

Mary learns the wine has been finished before the wedding celebration is over and informs Jesus. He explains to her that His time— meaning His time to perform miracles—is not yet. But thanks to God's release and Mary's encouragement, Jesus performs His first miracle, making wine out of water to save the reputation of the wedding couple. Three years after this first miracle, Jesus is crucified. Mary watches as Jesus, the Son of God but also her son, is brutally beaten and nailed to a cross. As He is dying in agony, He tells His mother and one of His disciples to care for each other like mother and son. Just as Mary loved and supported Jesus, He loves and takes care of her on the worst day of her life. Little did Mary know three days later, she would see her beloved Son again (Luke 24:1–10).

1. Why do you think Mary dismisses Jesus's words at the wedding when He says His time is not yet? How often do you encourage others?

2. After pondering in her heart all she has heard about Jesus, Mary speaks out at the wedding. Why do you think she chooses this time? How do you decide when to allow a difficult situation to play out on its own and when to intervene or ask for help? Have you ever regretted not saying something when it may have alleviated someone's problem?

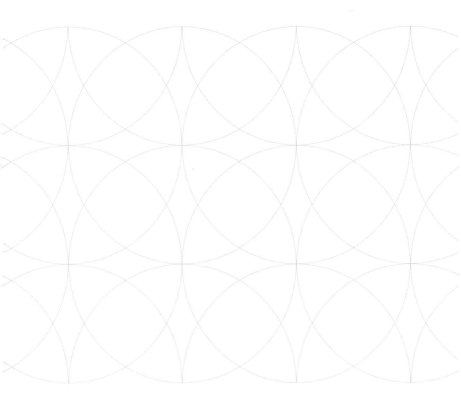

Day 7: Reflect and Take Action

KEY INSIGHTS

- God looks in the hearts of people (1 Samuel 16:7). He sees Mary's heart, which is full of humility, practicality, and agreement. What does God see when He looks into your heart?

- Mary puts together her ponderings and the prophesies she heard in her heart. It appears God utilized Mary to encourage Jesus to fully step into His calling at the wedding in Cana.

- Mary teaches us to be resilient in the face of difficult circumstances beyond our control, like when she has to walk a long way while pregnant and give birth near animals.

ACTION ITEMS

Think about what it means to see a miracle. Is it something spectacular or impossible, like changing water into wine? Or is it a matter of perspective? This week, focus on finding the miraculous, both big and small. Faith grows when we see God at work.

A lot can happen in three days. Mary experiences distress when losing Jesus at age 12 and grief at His death, and in both circumstances she feels joy three days later when she sees Him again. Life ebbs and flows with circumstances and emotions. If you or someone you care about is going through a difficult time, pray and ask God for the day of joy to come.

Mary remains calm throughout this passage. She is able to hold on to what the angel Gabriel told her as an anchor to weather the storms. Memorize a promise of God that you can stand on to help you remain calm when life is hard. 1 Peter 5:7 is a helpful one to get you started.

MARY MAGDALENE: CALLED BY NAME

Daily Readings

Day 1: Luke 8:1–2

Day 2: Luke 8:3, Luke 10:25–37

Day 3: John 19:23–25

Day 4: Luke 23:50–56, Luke 24:1–12

Day 5: John 20:11–15

Day 6: John 20:16–18

Day 7: Reflect and Take Action

This week we meet Mary Magdalene. Her story takes place early in Jesus's ministry, and although we do not know a lot about her, what we do know is significant.

Mary Magdalene meets Jesus in unusual circumstances. Scripture tells us she is possessed by seven demons. Jesus delivers her from the demons, and she becomes His follower. She finances His ministry, but the source of her wealth is never revealed.

Mary Magdalene appears at key moments in the life of Jesus. At the crucifixion, she is present to support Jesus and His mother, Mary. Afterward, she's one of the women who goes to the tomb to prepare His body. When she arrives, Jesus has risen to life and speaks to her.

Although Mary Magdalene is a quiet person, we see her being healed, as well as not only supporting Jesus's ministry financially but also following His teachings by becoming a disciple. She is devoted during His life, at His death, in grief, and in His life again as the first person to see Him after He is resurrected.

Mary Magdalene lives a tortured life possessed by demons, and Jesus sets her free. Although most of us have not been possessed, all of us can relate to difficulties in life, as well as the freedom we feel when the difficulties are lifted. Mary shows us what devotion looks like even in the darkest times.

Day 1

Freed by Jesus
Luke 8:1–2

Jesus's ministry is in full swing: He is teaching about the Kingdom of God, healing sicknesses, and casting out demons. He has His 12 male disciples, as well as some female ones, including Mary Magdalene.

Mary comes into this story quietly, but she's mentioned by name. "Magdalene" was not a family name but rather identifies that she was from Magdala, a thriving city about three miles north of Galilee. When Mary Magdalene meets Jesus, she's possessed by seven demons, a condition that undoubtedly wreaks havoc on her emotional, spiritual, and physical health. Mary Magdalene is a prisoner of suffering until Jesus, the Son of God, frees her. Mary Magdalene is now able to make decisions and take care of herself, and she chooses to follow Jesus, who saved her.

Most of us can relate to the need to find safety and refuge in certain areas of our lives. Not all Christians are able to find refuge in God when in distress. Sometimes we do not know how to do so, or God feels distant when we are struggling. But Mary Magdalene shows us that devotion and learning about God can bring us close to Him no matter what the circumstances.

FOR REFLECTION

1. When Jesus saves Mary Magdalene, she uses her newfound freedom to follow Him and celebrate His teachings. What are some of the biggest obstacles in your life right now? What would you do if someone took them away?

2. What has God placed in your life to help you feel whole when you're also feeling fragmented and broken?

3. Mary Magdalene is known to us by her first name and the city she was from. Think about where you're from or where you are at, not physically but spiritually. What would your new name be? What would you want it to tell people about you?

Day 2

The Giver
Luke 8:3, Luke 10:25–37

We know Jesus traveled all over teaching about the Kingdom of God, and He had no home (Matthew 8:20). Several disciples traveled with Him most of the time, so they needed a common purse to pay for food and other expenses.

Scholars say Mary Magdalene did not appear to be married or have a job. But she seems to have wealth, and she helps support Jesus, who gave back her life. Freed from affliction, she chooses to contribute to a cause she believes in.

In Luke 10 we read about the Good Samaritan, who saves a man beaten and left for dead and donates money to help him recover. Like the Good Samaritan who saves a stranger through his kindness and finances, Mary Magdalene gives to Jesus's ministry, enabling the disciples and Jesus to heal and help strangers.

In the time and place of Mary Magdalene, it was difficult for women to be independent and hold their own wealth, so it was especially generous for Mary and other women to donate their resources. She's a great model for us to contribute to ministries we believe in.

FOR REFLECTION

1. We learn how Mary Magdalene was similar to the Good Samaritan, but how was she similar to the man who was left for dead in that same story? Can you think of a time when you played a Good Samaritan role and when someone else did so for you? Describe what it felt like in each case.

2. Supporting Jesus's ministry makes Mary Magdalene a functional part of their society. People often contribute time and money to support ministries, but these methods exclude people who may not have the means. What are some other ways you can support a ministry?

| Day 3

Loyal and Loving in Grief
John 19:23–25

Mary Magdalene must have witnessed much during the ministry of Jesus, but nothing could have prepared her to be standing near the cross as Jesus was crucified, especially as many other disciples give in to fear and vanish (Matthew 26:56). Her savior had saved her life, but she can not save His.

What would it have felt like? Mary Magdalene had witnessed Jesus heal and change so many people, and now she stands with two other women, both named Mary. All of them loved Him but could not help

Him. They could only mourn, watching the cruel Roman soldiers play lots to win His clothes as He was dying.

It is heartbreaking to think of the immense grief Mary Magdalene must have felt watching our savior being tortured. Yet we also watch her be loyal, fearless, and loving toward Jesus to the end, standing next to Him on that unspeakable day. Most of the apostles fled, including Peter, who denied knowing Jesus three times. Mary Magdalene and the other women who stayed by His side demonstrate a deep connection and unrelenting devotion to Jesus that serves as an inspiring example to us all.

FOR REFLECTION

1. Why do you think many other disciples leave Jesus when He is caught and taken to the cross? Can you think of a time in your life when you weren't as brave as you wanted to be? What would you do differently?

2. Do you think there is a significance that three women named Mary stood together next to the cross? Do you think they drew strength from one another during this painful time? Who do you want standing with you when you have to go through an upsetting experience?

Day 4

Preparation Day
Luke 23:50–56, Luke 24:1–12

Mary Magdalene and the other women who witness Jesus die follow to see where and how He is laid to rest. Because it was Preparation Day (for Passover), as well as the day before Sabbath, they begin preparing burial spices and ointment to bring to Jesus's body on Sunday.

On Sunday morning, Mary Magdalene and other women go to prepare Jesus's body, but they find that the heavy stone that had been placed in front of the tomb has been rolled away, and His body gone. Two angels appear and tell the women that Jesus has risen and is no longer dead. The disciples do not believe the women's story—except Peter. But Mary Magdalene has hope and wonder building in her heart.

Mary Magdalene is with Jesus when He dies, and she is one of the first to learn of His resurrection. What do you think of these details, which point to something significant? Mary Magdalene's devotion is rewarded, showing us that loyalty is essential to staying close to God no matter what the circumstances.

FOR REFLECTION

1. Why is it important for the scriptures to tell us Mary Magdalene and the other women follow Joseph of Arimathea to the cave where Jesus is buried? Do you think that aside from practical considerations, anointing the body with oil and spices helped with the grieving process? Are there any rituals you turn to when you're feeling grief or pain? Do they include other people?

2. How does Preparation Day for Passover parallel the preparation in Mary's heart when she arrives at the tomb?

Day 5

Talking to Angels
John 20:11–15

In the Bible, the resurrection story is written differently in each book of the gospels. Just like eyewitness accounts from multiple witnesses, each version has variations.

In this passage, we see Mary Magdalene back at the tomb of Jesus. She's so sad that she doesn't realize she is talking to angels. She asks a stranger outside the tomb if he knows where Jesus is, not realizing it is Him.

Grief and sorrow are beastly, as we see in Mary Magdalene. She is unable to recall Jesus's words that He will rise after He dies. She is unable to process the angels sitting in His tomb. All she knows is her savior and teacher is gone. Her faith has diminished and sadness has taken over, but not for long.

FOR REFLECTION

1. Can you relate to Mary Magdalene's grief? All she wants is to be near Jesus, even in His death. The heartache she feels is something none of us want to experience. During dark times in our lives, we can feel distanced from Jesus, empty and longing for His comfort. Search for Jesus, like Mary Magdalene did. Look for Him especially when you feel disconnected. He is right there in front of you.

2. In her grief Mary Magdalene concludes that yet another terrible thing has occurred, that the body of Jesus has been taken away. Have you ever had a low moment when things just seemed to keep getting worse? How did you get through it?

3. Mary Magdalene has an encounter with angels. How is her reaction to them different from what you might expect if you saw an angel? Have you ever met someone who turned out to be an angel in disguise? Have you ever played an angel-like role for someone else?

| Day 6

Love Is Alive
John 20:16–18

Mary Magdalene encounters angels, but it doesn't register because sadness has clouded her reason. She sees Jesus and mistakes Him for a gardener. She is a mess and feeling hopeless.

Until she hears her name.

"Mary."

She instantly knows it is Jesus! She grabs hold of Him and does not want to let go. But because He has not ascended to God yet, she must release Him. She leaves Jesus to tell the other disciples that Jesus is alive and ascending to their Father God.

Love, joy, hope, and wonder must spill out of Mary Magdalene as she embraces her teacher, savior, and friend, Jesus.

Have you had this close experience with Jesus, feeling Him near you? Not all Christians have. Imagine what it would have been like to encounter Jesus like Mary Magdalene did. How would you feel if you heard Jesus calling you by name? We know it will happen one day, when we get to heaven. But let's also pray to have some kind of encounter with Jesus on earth, whether through others, by reading scripture, or by feeling a sense of His love for us.

FOR REFLECTION

1. Feelings and circumstances can change in an instant. At the beginning of this passage, Mary Magdalene is beyond distraught, and a few moments later she is beyond joy. Can you think of an occasion when you experienced disappointment immediately followed by relief or joy?

2. When Jesus first speaks to Mary Magdalene, she does not recognize His voice. Why do you think hearing her name allowed her to realize it is Jesus?

3. Sometimes in our pain we can't see the good things in our life or understand that a better change is coming. What do you do when someone you love is suffering too much to understand that things will get better? How do you reach them without minimizing their distress?

Day 7: Reflect and Take Action

KEY INSIGHTS

- Mary Magdalene shows her devotion and commitment to Jesus by being with Him near the beginning of His earthly ministry until His last day in His earthly body.

- Even though Mary Magdalene follows Jesus, she has doubts because of witnessing the trauma of the crucifixion. In grief, she forgets what He told her about dying and rising on the third day.

- Jesus calls Mary Magdalene by her first name when He sees her after the resurrection, suggesting a personal, friendly connection. Do you feel you have a personal, friendly connection with Jesus?

ACTION ITEMS

Mary Magdalene receives ministry from Jesus to get rid of the demons. Have you have had someone pray for you? Ask for prayer from a friend or at church, or call a prayer hotline.

Ministries rely on donations so they can provide needed services. Mary Magdalene recognizes this and donates to Jesus's ministry. Find organizations that mean something to you and donate any amount. If you have a hard time finding charities, here are some I trust and support: MendingTheSoul.org, FuelTheMission.org, HuggaBears.org.

When Mary Magdalene hears Jesus say her name, her entire world changes. Hearing your name in scripture can be powerful. Create a note card for yourself with a personalized scripture passage. For example, Romans 15:13: *May the God of hope fill you (insert your name) with all joy and peace in believing, so that by the power of the Holy Spirit you (insert your name) may abound in hope.*

MARTHA: THE SISTER WHO CALMED DOWN

Daily Readings

Day 1: Luke 10:38–39
Day 2: Luke 10:40–42
Day 3: John 11:1–4
Day 4: John 11:5–15
Day 5: John 11:17–27
Day 6: John 11:38–44
Day 7: Reflect and Take Action

After last week's account of the resurrection, we're backtracking to the time when Jesus was at the height of His ministry. Right before we meet Martha, we learn that Jesus had 72 disciples whom He sent out ahead to heal the sick and tell everyone that the Kingdom of God was near.

As Jesus and His disciples enter the village of Bethany, Martha invites Him and His disciples into her home. While Martha is working hard to prepare food for everyone, her sister is not helping. It sets up a conflict that

Jesus resolves in an unexpected way. Later in Martha's story, she asks Jesus for help with her brother, Lazarus. His response changes her faith.

Martha is a hard worker who initially seems to have a difficult time relaxing and prioritizing what's really important. She also has faith, which wavers when hard times come her way, but she regains it following a profound miracle. Martha is a practical realist who learns what living is all about when she encounters Jesus.

Martha is a model for the workaholics among us. It's easy to get caught up in the drive to be constantly busy, not giving yourself time to learn and think about spiritual matters. Jesus teaches Martha lessons about putting away work and focusing on listening and learning that can be applied to anyone who has a tendency to overdo it.

Day 1

Welcoming a Stranger
Luke 10:38–39

After teaching the Good Samaritan story, Jesus and His disciples go to the village of Bethany, where Martha greets Jesus and welcomes Him into her home.

Martha has a sister named Mary. When Jesus starts teaching, Mary leaves Martha and sits at Jesus's feet to listen. This action sets up a contrast between Martha and Mary. Martha is the greeter, the leader, and the hostess who welcomes Jesus into her home. Conversely, Mary is almost childlike as she sits at the feet of Jesus and neglects her household duties.

The scripture states that Jesus is welcomed by Martha into *her* house, which indicates Martha is the matriarch. She shows us the importance of greeting and welcoming Jesus, who was a stranger, into her home.

If Martha had not been so practical and welcoming, Jesus would not have had a place to teach and eat. We saw with Mary Magdalene that Jesus and His disciples depended on outside resources, so Martha's hospitality is a blessing. But sometimes it's easy for a busy host to forget the purpose of all those practical arrangements.

1. Are you more of a practical, organized person like Martha, or do you tend to gravitate toward the spiritual like Mary? What are the strengths and weaknesses of each tendency?

2. How do Martha's actions of greeting and welcoming Jesus into her home relate to how we can welcome Jesus into our home, also known as our heart?

Day 2

Bold for the Wrong Reasons
Luke 10:40–42

As the visit by Jesus and His disciples continues, Martha becomes angry because she has no help serving her guests. She is so upset that she goes straight to Jesus, who is teaching everyone, and asks if He cares about her because she has no assistance from her sister. She clearly wants Jesus to make Mary help her.

Jesus responds not by addressing the issue of serving per se; rather, He addresses Martha's anxiety. He tells her she's troubled by many things, when really only one thing is necessary: not her cooking and serving or Mary helping, but what Mary has chosen to do, which is to listen to His teachings.

Martha is bold to ask Jesus if He cares she is serving alone and to request Him, the guest of honor, to make Mary assist her. But Jesus sees stress as the source of this boldness and gently puts Martha on the right path. Many of us can relate to Martha in this story. We all have moments when we get frustrated with someone else, even though we are the ones causing our own drama.

FOR REFLECTION

1. Why do you think Martha asks Jesus to intervene instead of directing Mary to help? When you're upset with someone, do you

ever find it difficult to confront them directly? When is it okay to seek a third party's help?

2. We learn that Martha's gift is serving. Read Romans 12:6–8, which explains biblical gifts. Consider if any of them resonate with you. Are you using your gift well?

Day 3

A Step Back
John 11:1–4

Some time has passed since Jesus left Martha's family. He's in Jerusalem teaching that He is the Good Shepherd and the Son of God. The religious leaders try to stone Him to death, but He miraculously escapes to the Jordan River, where John the Baptist has baptized others. Once there, people come to Him realizing everything John the Baptist said about Jesus is true, and they believe Jesus is the Son of God.

Jesus then leaves to be with His disciples, where He receives word from Martha and her sister that their brother, Lazarus, whom Jesus loves, is ill. Jesus explains to His disciples it is not the end for Lazarus. Instead, God and Jesus will be glorified through Lazarus.

Martha and her sister do not ask Jesus to come to them; instead, they inform Him about Lazarus's situation. They expect He will do something to help. Notice the contrast to when Martha was in the kitchen, demanding Jesus make Mary help her. Martha has learned to take a step back and let Jesus take the lead.

FOR REFLECTION

1. English has just one word for all types of love, but Greek has four: *phileo* is friendly bond; *storge* is empathy bond; *eros* is romantic love; and *agape* is God's unconditional love. How many of these different feelings do you experience in a typical day?

2. How is Martha's message to Jesus about Lazarus different from when she speaks to Him in her home? How is it the same?

3. How do you ask people for help? Do you assume your friends will act if you share the problem, or do you need to ask directly? Is one way better than the other?

Day 4

No Condemnation
John 11:5–15

Scripture says Jesus loved Martha and Mary, but in the context of *agape* (God's love), not like His *phileo* (friendly) bond with Lazarus. Nevertheless, Jesus decides to wait two days before He goes to them. Jesus explains to His disciples that Lazarus has fallen asleep, and He will go to wake him up.

The disciples do not understand that Jesus means Lazarus has died, so Jesus explains it to them in plain words. Jesus also states that for their sakes He is glad He was not there when Lazarus died so the disciples would believe in Him. In yesterday's reading we learned that Martha is confident in Jesus's love for Lazarus and expects Jesus to help him when he is ill. Today we learn that Jesus indeed loves not only Lazarus, but also Martha and her sister. He does not condemn or redress Martha's anxiety and bossiness during His visit to her home. Instead, He has God's love for her.

FOR REFLECTION

1. What is the difference in the type of love Jesus has for Martha and for Lazarus? Why does this distinction matter? Do you feel God's love for you?

2. Why do you think Jesus chooses to stay two more days before He leaves to help Martha and her sister (review John 11:4)? When have you seen Jesus intervene in your own life, but in His timing, not yours?

| Day 5

Grief and Doubt
John 11:17–27

Jesus and His disciples make the journey to Bethany and find that Lazarus has been buried for four days. When Martha greets Jesus, we can hear her disappointment as she states that Lazarus would have lived if He had come sooner. But Martha also declares that God will give Jesus whatever He asks for.

Jesus tells Martha that Lazarus will rise again, and she jumps to the conclusion that He is referring to the last day. Jesus corrects her by explaining He is the One who brings resurrection and life. Martha agrees, not comprehending the miracle about to take place. Grieving, Martha believes but does not understand the power Jesus brings as the Son of God. In her mind, Lazarus could have been saved only if Jesus had come before his death.

Martha is one of the most "ordinary" of the women in this book. She was not proselytizing or present during other times in Jesus's life. She's not visited by angels. She's not called to a certain role. Instead, she is simply living her life, and Jesus becomes part of it. In this regard, I think many of us can identify with both her doubts and her faith.

FOR REFLECTION

1. Martha did not have hope that a miracle would happen. What do you do when you feel like a bad situation is hopeless?

2. In Martha's grief, she is not able to understand what Jesus is telling her. How often do your feelings get in the way of understanding the Word of God?

| Day 6

Unbound Faith
John 11:38–44

After Jesus speaks to Martha, they go to Lazarus's tomb. When Jesus orders the heavy stone to the tomb to be removed, Martha interrupts, stating there will be an odor from her brother's body decaying. He reminds her if she believes in God, she will see the glory of God.

Jesus commands Lazarus to come out of the grave. He does! His hands and feet are bound together for burial, and Jesus commands they unbind him.

Martha had allowed her doubts to bind her up, much like her brother was bound up in burial. But like Lazarus being unbound and freed from death, Martha is free to leave behind her preconceived notions of what is practical and walk in faith.

FOR REFLECTION

1. What does Martha's interruption at the tomb tell us about her thoughts? How can you remind yourself that God is active in your life?

2. How was Martha's faith unbound in this passage? Have you had moments in your life where your faith suddenly blossomed? Or have you built your faith more gradually?

Day 7: Reflect and Take Action

KEY INSIGHTS

- Martha's welcome to Jesus in her home is a nice example of how we can welcome Jesus into our hearts (Ephesians 3:16–17 and Revelations 3:20).

- Jesus looks past Martha's behavior and considers the root issues in her heart, which are anxiety and worry (Proverbs 21:2). It's important that we don't get so caught up in the practical necessities of life that we forget about our spiritual needs.

- Martha had head knowledge about Jesus and who He was, but when grief hit her, she had no heart knowledge of truly believing in what Jesus could do. How often does that happen to you? How can you move head knowledge into your heart?

ACTION ITEMS

Does Jesus live in your heart? If you accepted Jesus as your Lord and Savior, He does! If He does not and you would like Him to, read Romans 10:9–10 and follow these directions: Get a study Bible, read it, and start attending a Christian church.

Small acts of kindness can be meaningful to someone you do not know. Each day this week, perform a small act of kindness when you are out. Maybe that means holding open a door for a stranger, donating some food to an unhoused person, or smiling and making small talk as you wait in line at the store or on a commute.

This week's study highlights Martha's anxiety. How do you calm yourself when you are stressed? Write out your ideas in your journal. If you do not have ideas, search for some online.

Martha was loved even though she had issues with stress and doubted the power of God. Many people feel they are not perfect enough for God to love them. How do you feel about that? Take some time to meditate on 1 Corinthians 13:4–7 and Romans 8:38–39. Then spend time in prayer.

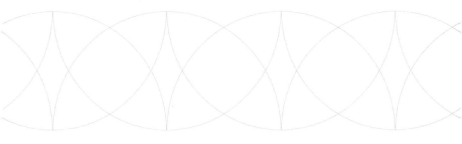

MARY OF BETHANY: THE SISTER AT JESUS'S FEET

Daily Readings

Day 1: Luke 10:38–39
Day 2: Luke 10:40
Day 3: Luke 10:41–42
Day 4: John 11:1–15, John 11:17–20, John 11:28–46
Day 5: John 12:1–3
Day 6: John 12:4–8
Day 7: Reflect and Take Action

Mary of Bethany is Martha's sister. Although we will cover much of the same scriptures from last week, this time we will focus on Mary's role. As we saw, she is the complete opposite of her sister. Rather than a practical doer, Mary likes to listen and connect. Her gift is not service, like Martha's; instead, she appears to have the gift of discernment.

Hungry to learn from Jesus, Mary of Bethany sits at Jesus's feet to learn from Him. She places listening to Jesus above listening to her sister. Jesus protects and defends Mary's activities twice because He says they are good choices. Mary of Bethany speaks little in the Bible, but her actions are huge.

Although Mary of Bethany has a different temperament from her sister, they feel the same about their brother, Lazarus. Like Martha, Mary grieves over her brother's death and has doubts when it seems Jesus did not arrive in time to help him. When life takes an unexpected painful turn, we can doubt God's care for us and become angry that He does not perform as we expected. Most of us will not be granted a wondrous miracle like Mary and her sister were, but we will learn from Mary's story that God will help us in unexpected ways, which often lead us back to Him.

Day 1

Learning Like a Child
Luke 10:38–39

We learned last week, in Luke chapter 10, that Jesus commissions 72 disciples to go out to heal the sick. They come back to report on the amazing miracles they have witnessed. Jesus then praises God for His will to reveal things to people who are not religious leaders. He refers to them as "children," meaning they are open to learning.

We meet Mary when Martha invites Jesus and His disciples into her home. Soon Mary of Bethany is sitting at Jesus's feet, listening to Him teach while Martha is busy serving. Mary wants to be as close to Jesus as possible, taking in every word He speaks. It brings us back to the image of Jesus praising God for revealing miracles to people who are like children (Luke 10:21). Mary exemplifies a girl leaning in and trying to understand the mysteries of God. She's very unassuming and humble about her desire to hear His word, simply positioning herself close to Him and listening to all He teaches.

This scene is another example of scriptures showing that women can be close to God and that they have pursued an understanding of Jesus's teachings from the very earliest days of His ministry on earth.

FOR REFLECTION

1. Mary of Bethany appears childlike as she sits and listens to Jesus, whereas her sister attends to "adult" matters like taking care of the guests. Do you ever find your adult ego getting in the way of seeking a better understanding of your faith?

2. We know how Mary's behavior differs from her sister Martha's in this passage. How are the sisters similar? In what ways do you possess qualities of both sisters?

Day 2

Positive Rebellion
Luke 10:40

Martha is working hard, cooking food and serving everyone because they are guests in her home. Mary becomes preoccupied by Jesus and His words. Yesterday we learned she is sitting at His feet. Mary will end up at His feet three times during this week's study. Being at someone's feet can connote reverence and servanthood. King David takes a similar position, sitting at God's feet in 1 Chronicles 17:16.

Martha grows angry about doing all the work by herself. She goes directly to Jesus, their honored guest, to try to guilt him into intervening and chastising Mary. Jesus points out that Martha is really trying to deal with her own worries. She is self-focused, but Mary is looking outward: rebellious in a good sense and hungry to learn.

Mary seems more sensitive than her sister when it comes to learning about spiritual matters. She steps out of her normal role, adjusting to an extraordinary situation without concern for her sister's demands. Martha is an adult, after all, who can make her own choices. Mary is not a people pleaser; she is more like a vessel wanting to be filled with the goodness of Jesus's teachings.

FOR REFLECTION

1. Do you think Martha would have felt better if Mary had explained her actions first? Have you ever left someone else to do more than their share of the work? Did you have a good reason?

2. Learning that Mary sits at Jesus's feet when there are other expectations of her shows us what kind of person she was. How do you see her? Can you relate to her choice?

Day 3

One Necessary Thing
Luke 10:41–42

Mary of Bethany is still at Jesus's feet, but Martha protests, believing Jesus will side with her. Instead, Jesus calls out Martha's anxiety and gently explains there is only one necessary thing to do, and Mary is already doing it.

Jesus takes what Martha says and turns it around for both Martha and Mary to hear. Jesus has Mary's back by rescuing her from Martha's expectations. He encourages Mary to continue what she is doing because it is the essential thing to do. He does not tell Martha what to do; instead, He only explains what really matters in the context of Him being in their home. Mary made the good decision, so there is no need to correct her. It does not matter if her usual role was to serve in her home. This occasion was not ordinary.

Mary models that no matter your age, your station in life, your role, or the expectations placed on you, it's essential to choose to listen to

Jesus's words and be in community with Him. Jesus teaches through Mary that spending time with Him is the most necessary thing.

1. Even though we still have not heard from Mary, Jesus defends her good choice to focus on Him at this dinner. Have you ever vouched for an unpopular choice that someone made, sticking up for them against criticism by others? Has anyone ever done so for you?

2. There's no sign that Mary protests or takes offense at Martha's attempt to shame her. How are Mary's actions stronger than words? Have your actions ever been stronger than words? What happened?

Day 4

In Grief, Doubt Spreads
John 11:1–15, John 11:17–20, John 11:28–46

Jesus is with His disciples when He gets notice from Mary of Bethany and her sister that their brother, Lazarus, is ill. Jesus explains to His disciples that they will wait to go to Lazarus because his death was meant to be a conduit for God's glory and for people to see Jesus was sent by God.

After Jesus returns to Bethany and speaks to Martha, she sends for Mary to speak with Him. Mary tells Jesus the same thing her sister did: that if He had been there, her brother would still be alive. She weeps at Jesus's feet. At this action, Jesus is deeply troubled in His spirit. He walks to the burial site and performs a miracle. Jesus raises Lazarus from the dead! After that, Mary and all who witnessed the resurrection believe in Jesus. How could they not?

When Mary first meets Jesus, she listens to Him teach. But in grief, while listening to her sister's doubt, she has difficulty holding on to her faith. The doubt Mary of Bethany shows toward Jesus in that moment is something we can all relate to, even if we've experienced miracles or felt close to God. As we will read tomorrow, Jesus does not hold anything against Mary or her sister for their doubt. Jesus loves us and is there for us even when we are upset or feel uncertain about Him.

FOR REFLECTION

1. Knowing Mary had listened so attentively to Jesus in her home, why do you think her doubt was stronger than her faith in Jesus? How does this account translate to modern-day Christians going through difficult times? When your faith is challenged, does it help to recall times when it was strong?

2. What does Mary weeping at Jesus's feet signify? How does it compare and contrast with her position during His first visit to her home?

3. Do you pray when you're feeling extreme grief or sadness? Why or why not?

Day 5

Listener. Doubter. Worshipper.
John 12:1–3

Soon after Jesus raises Lazarus from the dead, religious leaders want Jesus killed. His time to die an earthly death is drawing near, and all the pieces are falling into place. Perhaps that is why Jesus returns to Bethany to spend time with this family He loved. It's a touching scene: Martha serves without complaint, the resurrected Lazarus sits with Jesus, and Mary of Bethany anoints Jesus's feet with expensive perfume, using her own hair to wipe them clean.

It seems a strange gesture to us. But at that time, when a guest arrived, a servant would remove the guest's shoes, wash their feet with water, and dry them off. Scripture tells us Mary used expensive oil ("nard" from the spikenard plant) to anoint Jesus's feet, likely after they were already washed.

This picture of Mary taking a servant's posture, connecting with Jesus in this way, shows us she goes from a listener at His feet, to a doubter at His feet, and now a worshipper at His feet. Most of us go through changes in our relationship to Jesus. His fondness for Mary reminds us that His feelings for us do not change, even if ours do.

FOR REFLECTION

1. How do you treat your guests when they come to your home? What do you do to show hospitality and help guests refresh?

2. Why do you think Mary chose to use expensive perfume to anoint Jesus, rather than just washing His feet with water? Why use her hair? Do you honor God with any simple but personal behaviors or rituals?

Day 6

Devotion through Action
John 12:4–8

As Mary of Bethany anoints Jesus's feet with expensive ointment, Judas Iscariot, betrayer of Jesus, tries to shame Mary for wasting money. He states that it would have been better to sell the expensive oil and give the money to the poor.

Jesus defends Mary a second time; as with Martha's criticism, He knows the truth behind the harsh words. In no uncertain terms, Jesus tells Judas to leave her alone, that she was not wrong. Jesus reminds Judas that the poor will always be around and in need, but He will not always be.

Judas's false concern for the poor is trumped by the honest devotion in Mary's heart. Mary chooses Jesus again, over the expectations of others, and she does not care that Judas tries to guilt or shame her. She knows what is right. Her quiet devotion shows in her actions, and it counters the empty words of her critics.

Learning to do the right thing no matter what the circumstances are what Mary shows us in her story. Listening to Jesus and honoring Him comes before everything else. How does this translate to modern times? How can you demonstrate it in your own life?

FOR REFLECTION

1. The number three in the Bible means harmony, completeness, and new life. What does it symbolize that Mary was at Jesus's feet three times, in three different situations?

2. What do you do to refresh your spiritual life when it feels stagnant? Where do you find inspiration?

3. How was Mary's decision to anoint Jesus's feet similar to what Christians do on the Sabbath?

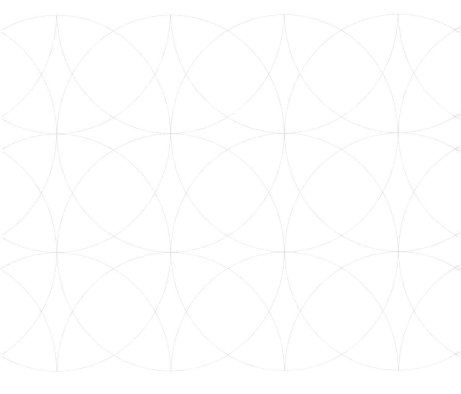

Day 7: Reflect and Take Action

KEY INSIGHTS

- Mary of Bethany is at Jesus's feet three times, in three different contexts. It is the closest she can be to Him in adoration, in grief, and in worship. She models that no matter what is happening in life, drawing close to Jesus is key.

- We hear Mary speak only once, when she tells Jesus she doubted Him. The other times we see Mary in action. These actions are what Jesus defends, showing us that actions can be stronger than words.

- Even though Mary doubts Jesus when Lazarus dies, Jesus does not hold it against her. He still loves her, and later defends her against Judas's criticism.

ACTION ITEMS

Focusing on Jesus can be challenging. What do you do to help you focus on God throughout your day? You might post a Bible verse on your car's dashboard or listen to soft worship music while working. List some ideas and try them out.

Many Christ followers would like to be near Jesus just like Mary of Bethany was. Try picturing yourself with Jesus, at His feet, or as in Psalm 23 with Jesus leading you to rest. Then speak your prayers when you see yourself with Him.

Washing someone's feet in the context of honor can be very special. Plan a gathering of family or friends to wash one another's feet to know how it feels. Finish with some scented lotion or some nard oil as a remembrance of Jesus.

THE SAMARITAN WOMAN AT THE WELL: TRANSFORMED BY LIVING WATER

Daily Readings

| Day 1: John 4:1–9 |
| Day 2: John 4:10–15 |
| Day 3: John 4:16–19 |
| Day 4: John 4:20–22 |
| Day 5: John 4:23–26 |
| Day 6: John 4:27–42 |
| Day 7: Reflect and Take Action |

The name of the woman in our final study has not been recorded in the Bible, so we know her as "the Samaritan woman at the well." (Although some denominations have named her Photina.) Whoever she was, she had a remarkable encounter with Jesus, who engaged her in conversation and treated her with a respect that signaled the universality of his ministry.

In the time of Jesus, Jewish people and the people of Samaria did not associate with one another because each thought the other was heretical. But the scriptures say that on this particular trip, Jesus "*had* to pass through Samaria" (emphasis added). Jesus arrives at a water well of particular significance, where he encounters the Samaritan woman of this week's study. Their encounter begins as He asks her for a drink of water, and the subsequent conversation encompasses so much more. By the end, the unnamed woman rushes into town to tell everyone that she met the Christ.

After being shunned by Jewish people, the woman at the well initially has a hard heart toward Jesus. He does not judge or belittle her but instead shares with her the good news of God. It moves her so much she has to spread the knowledge of who Jesus is.

It's not hard for us to find a connection with this woman at the well. She has bitterness in her heart; in her case it was because of religious persecution. Most of us have had bitterness grow within us when we've been misunderstood or disrespected. But when Jesus enters the picture and is understood for who He is, bitterness can melt away.

Day 1

A Drink of Water
John 4:1–9

Jesus has just left John the Baptist and is headed toward Galilee with His disciples. He has to walk through Samaria instead of going around it. The Samaritans and the Jewish people considered each other heretical and hated each other. Jesus ends up in Shechem, at a Samaritan well that Jacob himself had dug centuries earlier because it was near where his favored son, Joseph, was buried.

While Jesus rests, a Samaritan woman comes to draw water. He asks her for a drink. The woman can tell Jesus is Jewish, and she is bothered by the fact that He is speaking to her. She questions why He is asking her, a hated Samaritan, for water.

Although both the Jewish people and the Samaritans had Israelite roots, they were divided by many beliefs. In this story, Jesus symbolically closes the division, opening a dialogue with a Samaritan at a well dug by Jacob, who, you remember, was renamed Israel by God and whose children made up the 12 tribes that became the nation of Israel. Jesus wants to connect to the Samaritan in this passage, just like He wants to connect to us.

FOR REFLECTION

1. What is the significance of Jesus asking the Samaritan woman for a drink? Do you ever sense Jesus wanting to connect with you? What does it look or feel like?

2. Why do you think Jacob's well is a fitting meeting place for Jesus and the Samaritan woman?

3. Do you go to any places that are symbolic in your heart for important events in your life? Do you collect objects that symbolize special moments?

Day 2

Living Water
John 4:10–15

Jesus draws the woman into conversation, making her curious about God, Himself, and the "living water" He mentions. "Living Water" refers to both a spring of running water, and later the Holy Spirit, which Jesus talks about in John 7:37–39.

Soon we see an interesting back-and-forth, with the Samaritan woman trying to teach Jesus about the well they're sitting at and trying to provoke Jesus by asking Him if He is greater than Jacob. Jesus brings their conversation back to living water—the water that He gives, which brings eternal life. Not knowing who she is talking to, the Samaritan woman is thinking literally, assuming the water in question will quench her actual thirst and save her a daily trip to the well. She finds herself in conversation with someone she perceives as a mortal enemy, yet she has no fear of Him.

1. How often do you read the Bible and feel confused about spiritual thinking? When you learn something new from the Bible that's not in your paradigm, what do you do about it?

2. The Samaritan woman has no fear of the "Jewish man at the well," whom she believed was a great enemy to her people. What does that tell us about her character? How do you feel about others who do not share your world or religious views?

3. Why do you think the Samaritan woman feels the need to educate Jesus on who built the well they were sitting at? Have you ever tried to exert your knowledge over others when you did not understand their point? Did it help or hurt the situation?

Day 3

A Crack in Her Hardened Heart
John 4:16–19

Now the conversation takes an unexpected turn. Asking Jesus for His living water to help quench her thirst, the woman is surprised when Jesus responds by asking her to retrieve her husband. Soon He's telling her details of her own life, which is knowledge He could not have possessed by earthly means.

By trying to educate Jesus about the well and Jacob, the Samaritan woman is showing her knowledge. Jesus bypassed her earthly knowledge with talk about living water, eternal life, and His acquaintance with her personal story. He got her attention.

"I perceive you are a prophet," she tells Jesus, her need to see things in reality now channeled in a new direction. Jesus's words crack her heart and allow the living water to start flowing in. Hearing Jesus recount details of her own life enables the Samaritan woman to bypass her usual filter and move toward a deeper understanding. Can you relate? Sometimes when we hear a sermon, we can feel like it was meant just for us. When that happens, it gets our attention, just like Jesus did with this woman.

FOR REFLECTION

1. What do you think about the fact that the Samaritan woman has five husbands? How would that change a woman?

2. The Samaritan woman can grasp only things she can see and experience. How did the picture of "living water" help her start to see the concept Jesus is talking about? What metaphors or parables in the Bible help you understand God, Jesus, the Holy Spirit, or heaven?

Day 4

Something Else Is Coming
John 4:20–22

Understanding Jesus to be a prophet, the woman at the well begins to lay out why the Jewish people and the Samaritans do not get along. Again, Jesus takes their talk in an unexpected direction. Instead of discussing the differences, He explains that soon arguments over places of worship will not matter because something else is coming. He is very clear that salvation comes from the Jewish people, but states there will be something else for both them and the Samaritans.

Arguing, like the Samaritan woman does, is a natural reaction to being on different sides of a belief system. I am sure we have all been there, with our stance and pride on full view. This woman is not unlike us in this aspect. But Jesus does not look at division. He instead brings hope that things are going to change. He can do it in all our lives if we read and understand His word. There is hope. There can be change for those who encounter Him.

1. Why do you think the Samaritan woman starts focusing on the differences between Jesus and herself? Do you tend to do the same when you encounter others with different beliefs? What can you do to find common ground instead?

2. Jesus ignores the bait, does not argue with the Samaritan woman, and focuses on the bigger picture. She would not have been used to this behavior. What does this interaction teach us as we encounter others with different worldviews than ours?

| Day 5

What She Didn't Know
John 4:23–26

Jesus goes on to explain how this new worship will take place. The Samaritans and the Jewish people will worship God not on a mountain or in a temple but in spirit and in truth.

It may have been too much for the Samaritan woman to comprehend. Almost dismissive, she responds that when the Messiah comes, He will tell her what she needs to know.

"I who speak to you am He," Jesus calmly replies.

The Samaritan woman grows silent. We can almost feel her mind reeling. This woman focuses on what she knows and believes. She knows the first five books of the Old Testament. She believes she is talking to a prophet. She knows a Messiah will come one day to explain things to her (from Deuteronomy 18:18–19). What she doesn't know is that she is speaking to the Messiah. Until this moment.

We all can get stuck in our ways of thinking. We see the world through the lenses of our environment, just like the Samaritan woman. When Jesus explained who He was, it must have taken her breath away. When we hear a praise song or sermon or read scripture we have not noticed before, it can have the same effect. It can be stunning.

FOR REFLECTION

1. How does the Samaritan woman's argument with Jesus demon-strate similar divisions in our churches today? What do you think of the different Christian denominations? Can you have healthy discussions with people about doctrines that differ from yours?

2. The Samaritan woman is dismissive when Jesus explains how things will change. How do her response and behavior relate to Christians today who are not open to learning more about God? How do you react when someone tries to expand your knowl-edge of the Bible in ways that may be different from what you were taught?

Day 6

Thirst in Her Heart
John 4:27–42

As Jesus tells the Samaritan woman who He is, His disciples return. The Samaritan woman has no response; instead, she leaves her water jar, rushing to tell everyone to come see the Man who knows everything about her life, wondering if He is the promised Christ.

Many townspeople believe at first because of the Samaritan wom-an's testimony. After He stays for a few days, many more believe in Jesus because they have heard Him themselves.

This Samaritan woman starts off with a hard heart, division in her speech, and a reality check of what she knew and believed. When Jesus tells her who He really is, her heart becomes soft and full of wonder. Division is gone, and mysteries unfold. This woman at the well brings many people to Jesus because she has a great thirst in her heart that He is able to quench.

The woman at the well is changed because of Jesus, and because of her transformation she is able to share her testimony with others. Many of us can relate. Examine your own life to see how God has changed your heart. Or perhaps you know someone whose testimony grabbed your attention. Jesus changes people.

FOR REFLECTION

1. Why do you think the Samaritan woman doesn't respond after she learns Jesus is the Messiah? What does her silence symbolize? When have you been left speechless after learning new information?

2. Why is it important for the scriptures to tell us the townspeople believed in Jesus as the Messiah even without the testimony of the Samaritan woman? Did you become a Christian because you believed it was the thing to do, or did you make that decision based on what you learned about Jesus?

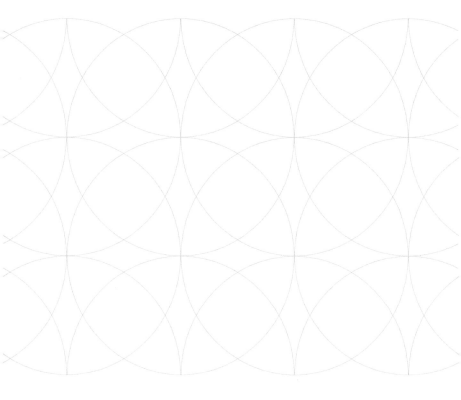

Day 7: Reflect and Take Action

KEY INSIGHTS

- We meet the Samaritan woman in the ancient city of Shechem, where God first appeared to Abram, Sarai's husband (Genesis 12:6–7). This place, plus Jacob's well, is a very significant setting for Jesus to meet the Samaritan woman.

- Jesus uses the image of a spring to help describe the living water He wants to give. He wants to help the Samaritan woman understand the difference between water you drink for thirst and His living water, which never leaves you thirsty.

- The Samaritan woman originally goes to the well to get water to quench thirst. Leaving her water pot behind indicates she has received the living water Jesus had for her.

ACTION ITEMS

To see a reenactment of this story, search on YouTube for the show called *The Chosen*, season 1, episode 8.

How is your heart toward Jesus? Pray and ask God to reveal any hard areas, then do a Bible study on what comes to mind. For example, if you feel misunderstood by God, search the Bible for discussions on how He knows you. A great passage for this purpose is Psalm 139.

A spring of water moves and bubbles out of the earth. A well of water sits without movement. Find a video or audio clip of spring (living) water and listen to it next time you pray to remind you of God's living water, which is the Holy Spirit in you when you accepted Christ (Ephesians 1:13–14).

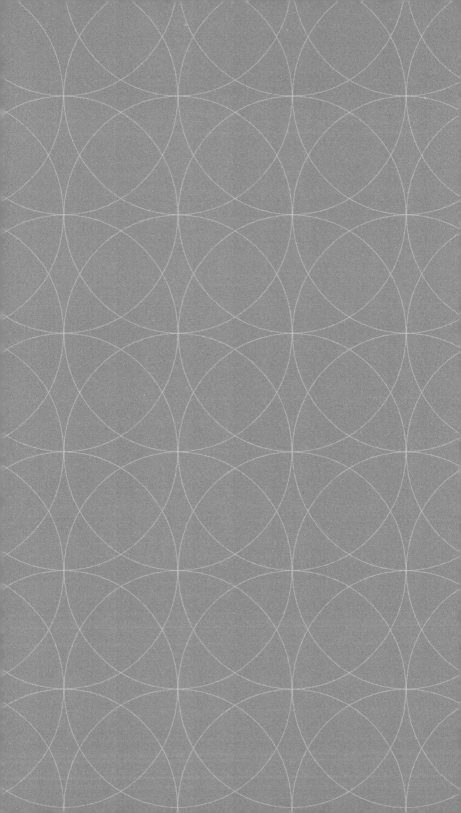

Group Study Guide

This Bible study is 12 weeks long, with six subchapters in each week. In a group study, each person should choose a subchapter for the week and come to the weekly meeting prepared to share their thoughts by answering a few or all of the following questions. Give everyone a chance to respond and encourage free discussion to continue for as long as time allows. Break up into smaller groups and institute time limits for discussions as needed.

1. How do you interpret these scriptures based on your research? What is the author trying to demonstrate through this woman?

2. Are there similar stories or scriptures that complement this particular woman's circumstances?

3. How did you answer the reflection questions?

4. Was there anything surprising about this woman or God/Jesus/ Holy Spirit in what you read?

5. Did you recognize any new revelations not mentioned in the commentary or insights?

6. Did you see God moving through the story? How?

7. What is your biggest takeaway from these scriptures?

8. How can you apply the characteristics or circumstance of this woman to your own life? What does it look like?

9. Which actions did you complete? Did they help you grow a little more with grace toward yourself or others and/or closer to God?

10. After reading the scripture and commentary, what will you do differently in your own life?

Index

Acknowledgments

I am thankful for the people who have done research, studied, and published their work, all of which helped me to understand culture, history, and the people of the Bible in order to honor the 12 women featured in this study. I am grateful for my amazing and hardworking editors, who had patience and kindness when I struggled to get my thoughts across. Most important, I thank God for His presence in so many details of my life over the years, including writing this book.

About the Author

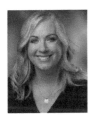 **Kimberlee Herman, MSW, LCPC,** is a Christian counselor, author, and speaker. She was a secular licensed therapist for many years but gave it up to be a licensed clinical pastoral counselor. She has a private practice in Phoenix, Arizona, and you can visit her website, RedeemedHopeAZ.com. Kimberlee loves to see God heal people and set them free from emotional and spiritual pain. She's the coauthor of *Wise Parenting: Guidelines from the Book of Proverbs.* In addition to writing and counseling, Kimberlee is a guest speaker at churches on various counseling and faith-based topics.